Embodying the Yoga Sūtra

for Lindy and Gail

and

for Peter

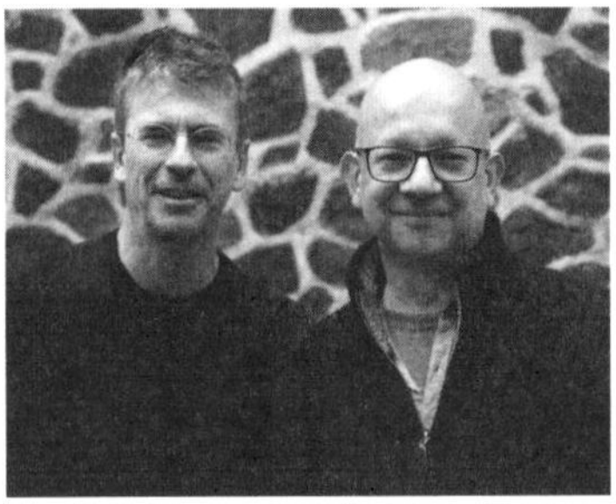

About the Authors

Ranju Roy and David Charlton are two of the most respected and well-loved yoga teachers in the UK today. In 2004 they founded Sādhana Mālā, an organisation that specialises in teacher training, study courses and retreats.

Together Ranju and David have produced and sold 13 booklets under the Funky Guru imprint; *Learning to Chant the Yoga Sūtra*, a set of 4 CDs; and have produced over 150 short video films for their bespoke online yoga training course.

Embodying the Yoga Sūtra is their first traditionally published book, part-funded by a successful Kickstarter campaign.

www.sadhanamalayogatraining.com

Embodying the Yoga Sūtra

SUPPORT ⊗ DIRECTION ⊗ SPACE

Ranju Roy and David Charlton

YOGAWORDS

Embodying the Yoga Sūtra: Support, Direction, Space

First published by YogaWords, an imprint of Pinter & Martin Ltd 2019

ISBN 978-1-78066-480-4

Also available as an ebook

British Library Cataloguing-in-Publication Data

A catalogue record for this book is available from the British Library.

Set in Adobe Text

Sanskrit calligraphy by Charles Cox
All illustrations by Ranju Roy

Printed and bound in the EU by Hussar Books

This book has been printed on paper that is sourced and harvested from sustainable forests and is FSC accredited.

Pinter & Martin Ltd
6 Effra Parade
London SW2 1PS

www.pinterandmartin.com

Contents

Introduction

Most students and teachers of yoga in the Western world will have come across Patañjali's Yoga Sūtra. Written about 2,000 years ago, this collection of 195 aphorisms has come to represent the foundation and pinnacle of the yoga tradition. The Sanskrit is dense, technical and brief: scholars across the world, and particularly since the late 19th century, have spent years analysing and interpreting their meaning. Yet, for the vast majority of today's students, the Yoga Sūtra has little relevance to their own practice. Most will not have read Patañjali's original text, and the various translations and commentaries in existence vary considerably in their emphasis.

Following the footsteps of our primary teachers – Peter Hersnack, Paul Harvey and TKV Desikachar – we believe that far from being an esoteric and academic text, the Yoga Sūtra is the key to transforming the way we *do* yoga. Each of these three extraordinary teachers illuminated aspects of the text and practice that brought an ancient teaching alive and made it fresh and contemporary. They moved it from the abstract to the practical: how it can affect the body (in āsana), the breath (in prāṇāyāma), the mind (in meditation), and the lived reality of our lives – in relationship to others. The Yoga Sūtra is a treasure trove of suggestions for both practice and for life. We set out to write a book that took this key principle – that the Yoga Sūtra is a *living* text – to explore how specific sūtras can deepen and change various aspects of our practice and our lives.

At the heart of our teaching is the concept of *viniyoga* – the appropriate application of techniques to the individual. One crucial aspect of our approach, arising particularly from Peter Hersnack, is the importance of *bhāvana* – images that play through your mind as you practise. In āsana and prāṇāyāma, how you place your thoughts is as important as where you place your limbs. Indeed *bhāvana* (which is sometimes translated as 'meditation') does not only happen sitting cross-legged with your eyes closed, but can infuse every aspect of your waking life. Our hope is that by understanding the meaning of the key yoga sūtras we present in this book, you may apply concepts such as these both 'on and off' the mat.

Most readers will be unfamiliar with many of the Sanskrit words and terms used, so we have tried to break these down etymologically to draw out the richness of association – the poetry, if you like – of the sūtras. Where we have kept to the original Sanskrit words, we have used italics and also diacritical markings. Please refer to the glossary for a discussion on some basics about Sanskrit and its pronunciation. Where words have become more commonly understood in English (for example, 'yoga', 'sūtra', 'āsana' and 'prāṇāyāma'), we have dispensed with the italics.

About the book

We begin each chapter with a single yoga sūtra (except Chapter 8, which has two), both in Devanagari and Romanised script, and then translated into English. A brief commentary on the sūtra follows, explaining some of the key terms. Each chapter then goes on to provide more context, both in terms of where the sūtra occurs – and in some cases, the sūtras preceding or following it – and how its teachings can be understood in our modern context.

There is no strict chronology to the chapters, nor are the sūtras in order, so the reader can dip in and out as they choose. The book is not a commentary on the complete Yoga Sūtra: there are plenty of excellent translations already available should you wish to study the whole text in detail.[1] Instead, over 16 chapters we have chosen to focus on 17 key sūtras which have immediate relevance to our practice. Further sūtras that relate to the main theme are then introduced and discussed in the body of each chapter.

There is no dearth of beginners' guides, resources and yoga courses available online and in bookshops. Rather than aimed at beginners, this book is intended for

1. We have included some important translations and commentaries of the Yoga Sūtra in the bibliography.

practitioners who are already familiar with the basics but would like to extend their knowledge of yoga to explore its history, philosophy and spiritual aspects, and how we might apply these in a modern context. We do not assume any prior knowledge of Sanskrit, however, and have endeavoured to keep the linguistic explanations as clear and straightforward as possible. For ease of reference, we have included a glossary of Sanskrit terms at the back of the book, alphabetised according to our standard Roman system.

Throughout the book, a common motif appears: the three terms that make up the subtitle: support, direction and space. This triumvirate was formulated by Peter Hersnack and coloured much of his brilliant and inspirational teaching. It is in many ways the most important touchstone for us. Only when you take support on something, can a direction arise, which in turn opens up a space – and a spaciousness – in your practice, and in your life. This image works, as you will discover through much of the book, both as a metaphor *and* as a lived, bodily experience. It is a common thread that runs throughout the whole book, in different ways in each chapter.

Each of the chapters concludes with a section entitled *Sādhana*. Here you will find specific practices and practical ideas that illuminate the chapter's primary sūtra. Some āsana sequences and poses are suggested, and in other chapters, we focus more on prāṇāyāma or meditative practices. Some chapters contain a lot of detailed information on the mechanics of practice, others are less elaborate, suggesting some simpler ideas to incorporate into your practice.

Sādhana is itself an important word. It is usually translated as 'practice' – but the connotations of the Sanskrit term imply a different, deeper and more fully engaged attitude towards whatever it is you are practising. *Sādhana* is the very means to perfection; it requires commitment, openness and faith – and a mindful attention to the present moment. It is the fundamental process which refines our very being.

When we set up our yoga practice, we thought long and hard about a name. A *mālā* is a rosary or necklace on which beads are threaded – you may have seen them worn by Hindu or Buddhist priests, or hanging outside roadside souvenir stalls in India – and we felt that nothing summed up better our aspiration to create a supportive, supporting, and profoundly connected circle of yoga practitioners than 'Sādhana Mālā'. Starting with a handful of students, this 'virtuous circle' has grown considerably, and many have gone on to become teachers, with students of their own. To all in the Sādhana Mālā family, we owe a debt of gratitude, not only for the financial support in crowdfunding the first edition of this book, but for the love, friendship – and sometimes patience and forbearing – that has got us this far.

Our yoga tradition is not static, handed down unchanged from one generation to the next like an antique or heirloom, but is alive and dynamic. We have received 'cuttings' from the '*sādhana* tree' nurtured by our teachers, and pass on our own 'cuttings' to students in the hope that they will take root and flourish in the future.

Ranju Roy & David Charlton
Sādhana Mālā
2019

Chapter 1

अथ योगानुशासनम् ।

Following the Path

YS 1.1 atha yogānuśāsanam

Now the instruction on yoga begins

The very first sūtra simply states Patañjali's aim: to present the authoritative teaching on yoga. Like all of the sūtras, it can be read simply at face value, as a straightforward statement of intent; or it can be unpicked and explored to reveal many other levels of meaning. The term *atha*, meaning 'now', is a traditional way to introduce sacred texts and conveys both authority and a sense of an auspicious beginning. It also suggests immediacy: "Now!" It is a call to action – to listen to and receive the teachings and to put them into practice. The phrase *yogānuśāsanam* consists of the words *yoga*, the subject under discussion, and *anuśāsanam*, an authoritative teaching that is passed on from one person to another. The choice of the word 'instruction' in our translation is deliberate here; instruction may be read as both a teaching and as something practical. The Yoga Sūtra is both: a teaching on the nature of being – and particularly the nature of mind – and an instruction manual on how to work with our minds to reduce our experience of fear, dissatisfaction and suffering.

The meaning of yoga

What do you understand by the term 'yoga'? Ask yourself, honestly: what does the word bring to mind? Physical postures, breathing exercises, meditation, philosophical ideas or a way of living? Perhaps a mixture of all these? Today, yoga is such a common term that we rarely stop to question what it means or where the word came from. For us, working within this tradition, 'yoga' is a technical term referring to something very specific, so let's start by exploring the word itself.

The entry for yoga in a classic Sanskrit-English dictionary[1] is one of the largest in the book and contains a multitude of definitions, many of which (on the surface, at least) have little to do with the practices we are discussing here. Even in the context of a practice system, yoga has been used to describe a wide variety of techniques and ideas over the centuries in India. When new yoga students begin to develop their interest in its history and ideas, it is common, and perhaps naively reassuring, to assume that yoga is a definitive, timeless and complete body of wisdom that has been transmitted faithfully without change since the dawn of time. In fact, nothing could be further from the truth. Although there are certain shared themes, there are very few (if any) ideas, definitions and practices common to all modern schools of yoga – let alone those that have flourished and faded over the course of history. The development of yoga is complex, and the proliferation of different forms of yoga in the West over the last 50 years has made it even more so. It is perhaps better to think of the term 'yoga' as a common word that has been used at different times and in different contexts to refer to quite different things.[2] This is particularly important if you are reading this book having studied yoga within a different tradition, and already have ideas about the meaning or significance of the word. It may be presented differently here, but that doesn't necessarily mean either definition is incorrect.

1. M. Monier-Williams, *A Sanskrit-English Dictionary* (Oxford: Oxford University Press, 1899).

2. Mark Singleton calls 'yoga' a *homonym* (a word with the same sound but with various different meanings), to indicate how yoga is, and has been, used at various times. Mark Singleton, *Yoga Body: The Origins of Modern Posture Practice* (Oxford: Oxford University Press, 2010).

The word is most commonly derived from the Sanskrit root[3] *yuj* meaning to 'link' or 'join together', in the sense of yoking two things together. Many Indo-European languages (including English) are related to Sanskrit, and thus the root *yuj* has a direct connection to the English word *yoke*. Because Sanskrit developed within an agricultural culture, many of its words have their origins in ideas associated with such a context. *Yuj* was originally used to refer to the yoking of two oxen together so that they could be used for ploughing, or to draw a cart. Two principles (in this case, the oxen) are connected in a way that allows them to interact to produce a useful outcome. When applied in a personal sense, there can be a yoga whenever an individual links themselves to something, or engages in a specific activity, in order to achieve a desired outcome. This principle applies almost universally to the contexts in which 'yoga' and other words derived from the root *yuj* are used, even in quite ordinary or mundane usages. Thus for example, yoga can be used in the context of putting on a suit of armour. By employing the armour, one gains a certain invulnerability to attack. Similarly, yoga can be used to describe a magic trick: performing a trick in the prescribed way produces the illusion of magic. Both of these are examples of the use of the word 'yoga' in a non-spiritual context.

In the context of yoga as a practice, or transformative process, this is perhaps the most universal principle and one we should not forget: in yoga, we place ourselves in relationship to something in order to produce a positive effect. We yoke ourselves to a practice, a discipline, an object of meditation, a yoga posture or a breathing technique in order to bring about a positive transformation. But: no relationship, no yoga. Similarly: no transformation, however small, no yoga. What we might link ourselves to, what type of practice we might engage in, and what techniques and qualities we bring to the practice, form the scope of the rest of this book.

3. It is a common strategy to identify the roots of Sanskrit words in order to understand their meaning. Some words can be derived from more than one root, so examining the possible roots of words is a traditional way to explore nuances and alternative meanings. The word yoga itself can be derived from more than one root (*dhātu*). *Yuj*, the most commonly stated root is given here; in Chapter 2 a different root will be suggested for the specific meaning of yoga in the Yoga Sūtra. Both are relevant and give us different lenses to explore the word at the heart of our story.

Yoga is frequently translated as 'union', but here, this is rather misleading. To us, 'union' suggests two things becoming one, whereas central to the idea of 'yoking together' is the fact that *the two things remain two things*. They are united only in the sense of being linked, and it is in their interaction and relationship that there is yoga, not in them merging together inseparably.[4] This, for us, lies at the very heart of yoga, and is fundamental to our approach to the subject – both as teachers and as practitioners.

Yoga as relationship: 'Taking support'

We have already suggested that the fundamental meaning of the term 'yoga' is to engage in a relationship with something to bring about positive change. But what are the qualities that we need to bring to this relationship? The short answer to this is that we need 'to take support' on whatever it is that we are linking to. 'Taking support' is a slightly awkward phrase, but it is useful. As the leading term in our subtitle, the question of support – what it is, where it can be found and how we take it – is crucial. It's worth spending a little time getting this cornerstone laid, since it, quite literally, supports everything that is to follow.

Think of how you use a walking stick. It is a literal 'support' that allows us to do something that otherwise might be difficult or impossible (assuming we have difficulty walking). So let us consider the steps (no pun intended!) in using the walking stick. First, you need to have an *intention*: the desire to walk better and to use the walking stick for support. Walking sticks don't pick you up – you have to take the initiative. The next step is *learning to use* the walking stick: there is some technique involved. Thirdly, you have to lean on the stick and *allow* it to support you. This may seem obvious, but in fact is a critical step in our analogy. Unless you actually lean on it, have confidence in its strength and stability, and really give yourself to it, it can't support you. Finally, you have to be *willing to accept* what it can give you in order to step forward. Using a stick may feel awkward or

4. In the Yoga Sūtra, *saṃyoga* is used to indicate a relationship where two things become confused as if one, with a consequent lack of freedom and vitality (YS 2.17). By contrast, yoga is a relationship where the difference between two principles is maintained and yet in their interaction there is vitality, mutual support and freedom. This is discussed in greater detail in Chapters 4 and 8.

unnatural at first: it takes practice to develop your technique and build a good working (or walking!) relationship with it.

We can use this analogy to understand the practice of yoga as 'taking support' or 'benefiting from a supportive relationship'. To do this requires the following steps:

- choose your support appropriately
- take the initiative to use the support
- learn the technique to engage with the support
- have confidence in the support
- let the support support you
- develop your technique or relationship with it through repeated practice

In modern yoga classes, 'supports' tend to mean equipment – blocks and belts, for example. In this context, however, supports could include: yoga postures, breathing techniques, meditation practice, the observance of certain disciplines, cultivating our relationship with the Divine, repeating a sacred word or phrase, adopting certain attitudes, or having a special relationship with a teacher. These and other such supports will be explored in the following chapters.

Tradition, teachers and transmission

In India, lineage and tradition are greatly valued. Teachings that are ancient and have stood the test of time are prized, and teachers in India are often at pains to emphasise the purity and longevity of their lineage. The oldest sacred texts, the Veda,[5] are said to contain everything that needs to be known and are considered to be the source for all orthodox spiritual teachings.[6] They are collectively classified as *śruti*, (literally, 'that which has been heard'), which means that they are understood as divine revelation – 'heard' in the deepest states of contemplation. All subsequent teachings are seen as elaborations, stemming from these most sacred roots. Although modern scholars and historians might take issue with such a claim, what is important here is the idea

5. There are four Veda, the Ṛg, Sāma, Yajur and Atharva, each a vast collection of sacred hymns. Different families and traditions trace their lineage back to one of these four texts. Their dates are very approximate, but scholars believe them to be roughly 3,000 years old, and certainly some parts are even older.

6. Traditionally, teachings arising from the Veda were called *sanātana dharma* (the Eternal Teaching). The term Hinduism was coined much later by the Persians and Greeks. Here, we use the term 'orthodox' to refer to teachings which accept the authority of the Veda. Buddhism is an example of an ancient Indian tradition which does not, and is therefore considered to be heterodox by the Vedic purists.

of the pure transmission from teacher to student from an authentic source.

The term *anuśāsanam* indicates that the teaching of the Yoga Sūtra is such a tradition. It has both authority and has been transmitted faithfully through *paramparā*. *Paramparā* (literally, 'from one to another') is a word used to indicate the lineage of the tradition and the key lineage holders. However, *paramparā* also evokes the idea that the teaching must be transmitted from one person to another in all cases. The human relationship is essential for effective teaching – it cannot simply be learnt from a book (such as this!). Thus we return to the idea of a supportive relationship, in this case the relationship between teacher and student. This relationship should allow the student to learn the ideas and practices offered by the tradition, and also to flourish and grow as their practice deepens. The *paramparā* from teacher to student is, therefore, another yoga (in the sense of relationship), and it is present in every teaching situation – from the mundane to the most profound. Through our lives there have been teachers at every stage, beginning with parents, teachers at school, mentors and colleagues at work... the list goes on. In the yoga tradition, the quality of the relationship between teacher and student, and the teacher's ability to discern what is appropriate and of value to the student, is acknowledged as one of the most important factors in making the practice effective.

Being present and committed to the truth

Atha – 'Now'– not only conveys authority and marks an auspicious beginning, it also suggests an immediacy and a presence in the here and now. It is a call to see things as they truly are without the colouring of the past or thoughts of the future.[7] A fundamental premise of yoga is that our minds are rarely clear lenses through which we encounter the world, but instead are full of distractions, memories and projections that colour our view of both the world and our place within it. The purpose of yoga is 'to clear the

7. The primary and earliest commentator on the Yoga Sūtra, *Vyāsa*, understands *atha* as representing *adhikāra*. *Adhikāra* indicates the authority of the teaching and Patañjali's authority to transmit this teaching. Our primary focus here, however, is on *atha* meaning 'in the present moment'.

lens' so that we encounter the world fully in the present, just as it is, without distraction or distortion. We could somewhat creatively say that the whole of the yoga project is encapsulated in the very first word of the Yoga Sūtra: *atha* – being entirely present and aware of what *is*.

Being present with a totally clear and stable mind is not easy, as anyone who has tried to meditate will know. Our minds are full of habitual patterns, memories, desires and fears, and countless concepts through which we make sense of the world. This is natural and what makes us human. However, all these thoughts and the feelings that arise in connection with them are also the source of much distress and misunderstanding about the true nature of ourselves and the world around us. The Yoga Sūtra presents a complex psychology to explain how our minds work and suggests that through practice we can make the mind more stable, more present and less distorting. Then we are less prone to distraction, less concerned with memories from the past or worries about the future, and we see ourselves and our world with more clarity. The payoff, Patañjali suggests, is that we will be able to live more peacefully and wisely, and reduce the distress in our lives. To be in a state of *atha*, moment to moment, is thus to be in a state of yoga.

'The Yoga Sūtra presents a complex psychology to explain how our minds work and suggests that through practice we can make the mind more stable, more present and less distorting.'

So how to begin such a journey? The answer is NOW. *Atha* demands that we put the teachings of yoga into practice, acknowledging the reality of where we are right now and being realistic about the steps we need to take. This requires us to 'pick up the stick', to commit to the practice and begin the journey from where we are. It also requires that we learn how to take some steps and choose the right supports for the journey – and this almost inevitably means that we will need a skilful teacher to help guide us on our way.

Sādhana: Learning to be still

To become fully present, we have to learn how to pay attention to ourselves. This 'paying attention' does not mean simply giving free rein to our various likes and dislikes, but instead requires us to become alive to the sensations within our bodies, the patterns of our breathing and, perhaps most importantly, the ever-changing contents of our minds. In modern life, with all its demands, variety and overwhelming sensory stimulation, it is easy to find ourselves simply responding to and negotiating the external world, with little attention to what is going on inside. But just as we move about in an external world of sensory input, we also have an inner landscape that we can explore. This inner landscape is a world of subtle physical sensations including many of our normally automatic processes, such as breathing and digesting. And then there is the bubbling cauldron of thoughts, judgements, memories, fantasies and emotions that we call the mind. Exploring our inner landscape may be a strange and unfamiliar process in the beginning. We may start by feeling or noticing very little at all. However, with practice, it becomes increasingly vivid and familiar. We can train our inner sensitivity. In a similar way we can learn to observe the processes that arise in our minds and, as we do so, we notice certain patterns of thought and behaviour that were previously unconscious.

This process of cultivating inner awareness is something that yoga shares with many other meditative disciplines. It is difficult if too much is happening around us, so it is usual to sit still in a quiet space where there are minimal distractions. It's tricky to watch a movie and focus on the details if the screen is unstable. By keeping the body still and our minds relatively quiet, it's as if the screen on which our personal movie is being projected is being held stable.

We may sit still in meditation, work with our bodies during a posture practice or focus on our breath during a breathing practice. In each case, we are cultivating our sensitivity to our inner landscape and processes. We generally start our yoga journey with the emphasis on postures and movements, but the intention is always to deepen our inner awareness. This is the primary reason why movements are performed slowly and smoothly, or postures are maintained for some time: it is easier to attend to subtle inner sensations, observe the breath, and notice thoughts and feelings that arise. For the same reason, the points in a posture practice where the body is still, between movements, are perfect places to cultivate such an awareness and *actually practise being still*. Therefore, a good starting point for our discussion of practice is to appreciate that *stillness is part of the practice*.

Being still is not easy, and for most of us it is an unfamiliar state – we react, respond and fidget our way through life. Beginners in a yoga class will often focus well as they are guided through a movement or posture but afterwards will rearrange their clothing, scratch an itch or look around the room. In doing so they easily lose

'A good starting point for our discussion of practice is to appreciate that stillness is part of the practice.'

their calm and focus and miss the opportunity to really experience the effect of what they have just done. Telling students to simply return to a point of stillness can make a big difference. This still point is an important part of the practice itself, and it takes discipline and awareness to actively resist 'scratching the itch'.

There are points of stillness throughout the practice. We use 'transition' postures as starting and completion points for the different postures; these can be used to practise stillness. We shall meet them in more detail in Chapter 3.

There is an important principle in cultivating stillness: we need a light touch. If we are making too much effort, or if there is tension in the body, being still can be exhausting and counterproductive. Can we be still without being rigid? Can we stand with a sense of lightness and stability with a minimum of effort? Although our principal goal is simply to notice and be with what is, this is also an opportunity to let go of any obvious patterns of holding and tension. It is usual to start a practice with a short period of *samasthiti* (assuming we are going to begin with standing postures), as a way to ground ourselves in the present moment – *atha* – as well as to orient ourselves towards what is to come. At times we could even extend this simple standing for a few minutes; it is surprising how challenging and yet grounding this can be. Similarly, it can be useful to stand for a minute or two at the end of the standing postures, as a way to experience what has changed through the standing work – listening to the resonance of the postures in the body. We can use still points for the other posture groups as well, such as kneeling after prone backbends, or resting quietly on the back for a few moments after a lying posture.

Samasthiti can also be used at the very end of a practice as another reference point. This is a little more unusual, but very useful as it gives us an opportunity to see how our basic standing posture has been changed through the practice. Such changes may be quite subtle, but again our awareness of the changes can become more sensitive with practice. We sometimes say that yoga can change both our sense of *being* (how we experience ourselves in the space that surrounds us), and our quality of *seeing* (how we perceive that space). Standing for a minute or so at the end of the practice can give us a moment to explore both, asking ourselves questions such as "How am I standing?", "How connected is my pelvis to my feet?", "How free does my head feel?", "Do things around me look more vivid?", "What sounds can I hear?". As we quieten the body and refine the senses, the contours of our inner landscape come into gradual focus, allowing us to explore our engagement with yoga ever more fully. Our *being*, the very way that we stand, has changed, and that changes our *seeing*. However modestly, each time we practise, we stand afresh, both present in the Now and linked to the ancient tradition of yoga.

Chapter 2

योगः चित्तवृत्तिनिरोधः ।

Yoga is a State of Mind

YS 1.2 yogaḥ cittavṛttinirodhaḥ

Yoga is directing and containing the activities of the mind

The second sūtra defines the term 'yoga' as used in the Yoga Sūtra. This sūtra has a special name: the *lakṣaṇa sūtra,*[1] so called because it states the essential characteristic of Patañjali's system. It is a technical definition of yoga that informs the text. There may be disagreement about what the word yoga means within a greater context (as we have explored in Chapter 1), but here there is little scope for debate once the definition is understood.

Yoga is defined as a state of mind: the term *citta* means 'mind' and in a state of yoga its nature is *vṛtti nirodha.* The word *vṛtti* comes from a root meaning 'to turn' and indicates that all mental processes are in a constant state of flux. This includes perceptions and our responses to them, thoughts, feelings, memories and so on. Anything that arises in our psychological and emotional arena can be described as *citta vṛtti. Nirodha* is a particular state of the *citta vṛtti.* In his commentary to the Yoga Sūtra, Vyāsa describes five basic states of mind, two of which are fundamental to yoga. Confusion about these levels has led to a lot of misunderstanding about the practice of yoga, and so we shall explore them below.

Of the two levels of *citta vṛtti* that are relevant to yoga, the first (and more accessible) Vyāsa calls *ekāgra* (one-pointedness). Here the mind is focused in a chosen direction for a period of time: it is a practice. The second level of *nirodha* (actually called *niruddha* by Vyāsa) cannot be practised in the ordinary sense; it may or may not arise. In *niruddha*, the containment of the mind is total and the *vṛtti* are said to be absent in that the mind appears to be completely still and clear. This state may arise in very deep meditation, but exerting effort 'to stop the mind' will not help to bring it about. It is very important to understand that the route to quietening the mind is to focus it, not to suppress it.

1. *Lakṣaṇa* means 'essential quality'; without it an object would be something else.

The word 'yoga' revisited

Although the word yoga is more commonly said to be derived from the Sanskrit root *yuj*, (as discussed in Chapter 1), there is an alternative root, *yuja*, which means 'to meditate' or 'focus on'. Vyāsa explicitly states that "Yoga is *samādhi*" (a deep state of complete meditative absorption), thereby indicating that *yuja* is the preferred root in this context. Therefore this should be taken as the root of the term 'yoga' as defined by Patañjali and is completely consistent with his definition of yoga as *citta vṛtti nirodha*. So why did we present the root of yoga as *yuj* in the first chapter? Our answer is that although *yuja* is the specific primary root applicable in Patañjali's very particular definition here, an exploration of yoga as 'linking' is fundamental to our discussion, and *yuj* yoga is therefore also relevant. Often in Sanskrit, a word can be derived from more than one root. The author or commentator may use a primary root to emphasise a specific meaning, but the other meanings (and therefore other roots) may also be important. Thus the primary meaning of yoga in YS 1.2 is *samādhi*, 'to meditate deeply on something'; while the secondary meaning is 'a link to allow the mind to come into relationship with a chosen object' so that the *citta vṛtti* become *ekāgra*, or one-pointed.

Citta, citta vṛtti and the nature of mind

Most of us spend a tremendous amount of time thinking. But not so many of us spend a lot of time thinking about thinking. What is thought? Where does it come from? What is its relationship to us? In the second sūtra, the *lakṣaṇa sūtra*, Patañjali defines yoga as a specific state of our *citta*, where *citta* is understood as 'mind'. Therefore, yoga is a state of mind.

The term *citta* is a very important word both in yoga and Indian philosophy generally. When we translate *citta* using an English word such as 'mind' we must be careful. Do we mean the same thing? Do our culturally specific associations with the word 'mind' add to or detract from the original? In this particular case, we should be clear that *citta* does not just refer to mind and cognition; it includes all psychological phenomena such as our emotions, feelings, perceptions, imagination, memories, reflections and, of course, thinking. Anything that arises within the field of our experience is part of *citta*, or to be more precise, *citta vṛtti*.

As already stated, *vṛtti* comes from a root meaning 'to turn' and so *citta vṛtti* are movements or turnings of the mind. Ideas, thoughts and memories arise, exist for some time and then slip away or transform into something else (another thought, feeling, or memory). *Vṛtti* captures the dynamic nature of our psychological content and furthermore it reflects the cyclical nature of thoughts and emotions. They revolve into and out of consciousness as we endlessly 'turn over' ideas in our minds.

There is a tendency in the West to create a division between head and heart, between thoughts and emotions. We might say "they are all in their head," or "they work from their heart," and we instinctively know the difference. Embedded in our language and culture is a division between thinking and emotional processes, as if they occur in different locations or are divorced from one another. This division is not present in the term *citta* – it includes all aspects of our experience. Yoga is sometimes misunderstood as concerning itself only with our cognition in a kind of dry, unemotional way, whereas in reality it includes the whole gamut of feelings, from happiness and joy to existential fear, desire, and even hatred.

Citta has a number of functions. It is a storehouse for memories, tendencies, and habitual patterns, and it is the instrument through which we perceive and digest information from the senses. It is also the cauldron in which we process our fantasies and anxieties. *Citta* is often described as the medium through which our consciousness operates, and what arises in the way of thoughts, feelings, emotions and memories can be seen as movements of the *citta,* rather like waves or ocean currents. The ocean is *citta* and the waves or currents, *citta vṛtti*. However, we shouldn't forget that the *citta vṛtti* are not fundamentally different to the *citta* itself, just as waves and currents are not fundamentally different to the ocean. Waves are movements on the surface of the ocean and clearly visible to the observer; currents are movements largely below the surface and harder to observe. In a similar way, there are *citta vṛtti* that we are conscious of (like the waves) and others we are not normally conscious of, like currents under water.

The Yoga Sūtra (and the philosophy of yoga generally) proposes a range of different terms and concepts to describe the contents of the mind and its forces and mechanisms. Although yoga is often thought of as a system of working with the body, the Yoga Sūtra is essentially a psychological treatise, fundamentally concerned with our mind. We may work with the body, and emphasise the primary role of the breath, but ultimately it is all to affect our state of mind. If there is no change in our mental state when we practise, there has been no yoga, no matter how beautiful or elaborate our postures.

Citta vṛtti and suffering

Traditional Indian philosophy addresses a central concern: the experience of human suffering and the means to reduce it. Yoga is no exception. It is important here to differentiate between physical pain and our experience of it, and the distress it causes. Similarly, when we consider anything that happens to or around us that causes us anxiety or distress, we must differentiate between what happens and the responses we have to it. Our experience of distress and suffering is often our response to our anxieties about, or anticipation of, distressing situations. In Sanskrit, this is called *duḥkha*. *Duḥkha* is conventionally translated as 'suffering', which is fine as long as we appreciate that we are referring to our psychological and emotional response to a situation (or imagined situation) and not the situation itself, which is frequently beyond our control.[2]

Yoga recognises that much of our suffering is a response to change on some level, either dissatisfaction with the past, an emotional response to what is happening in the present or anxiety about the future. The very process of dissatisfaction implies movement in the mind, in other words *citta vṛtti*. We respond to and evaluate perception, consider the potential implications of things, or simply turn over thoughts and worries in our head. 'Turning' perfectly describes what happens when we become worried about something; the 'anxiety track' is stuck on repeat. Our experience of suffering is inextricably linked to the process of change and movement in our minds.

By contrast, when the mind is focused and stable, particularly when the direction or object of focus is supportive (i.e. not a source of worry), then we are not suffering. We are simply focused on something that is not a cause for distress. The *vṛtti* that might be concerned with dissatisfaction, fear, anxiety and so on are absent during such moments of focus. It would be a mistake to think that *vṛtti* are not present at such times, as the mind is still active, but during this state all the *vṛtti* in the mind are focused on the supporting object and disturbing *vṛtti* are temporarily absent. It's as if we have some time off for good behaviour – here our 'good behaviour' is temporarily stabilising the mind on a good support. There could be many directions of focus that can act as a support, but in this approach, the prime example is the breath.

If stabilising our minds on a good support can temporarily relieve our experience of suffering, what happens afterwards? Are we back to square one? Anyone who has done an effective yoga practice, even in a basic class, knows the answer to this: no! We do not return to the place we started from. Even if nothing appears to have changed, we generally feel in a place of renewed strength as if we have had respite from our suffering. Often, we feel as though the situation that has been bothering us has reduced

2. See Chapter 4 for further exploration on the nature of *duḥkha*.

in size and the disturbing *vṛtti* similarly diminished. This 'perspective reset' allows situations that may have grown out of all proportion to return to their proper place and consequently we feel more at ease.

The Yoga Sūtra explains this process.[3] It identifies five fundamental forces that cause us problems, called *kleśa*[4] (literally 'that which afflicts'). All are said to come from a fundamental misunderstanding about the nature of ourselves, and particularly our minds, and an inability to accept the reality of our situation. The *kleśa* exist in us like dormant seeds, becoming active only when circumstances trigger their growth – something or someone 'pushes our buttons'. Then they grow like shoots. While small, they may be manageable, but they can get stronger until they overwhelm us. When fully aroused, they are almost impossible to overcome until they begin to subside. However, most of the time we experience distress in varying levels of intensity, which we can work with. The practice of settling the mind on something else gives both a relief from the disturbance and an opportunity for the *kleśa* to settle so they return to a manageable level.

When we are really bothered about something it can be difficult to reorient the mind and in such circumstances our attempts to focus on our practice can feel frustrating. Fortunately, it is not an all-or-nothing process. Making the attempt, however incompletely, does make a difference and usually, by the end of the practice, there is some shift of perspective. Thus, another useful definition of yoga here is 'reaching a new state' or 'effecting positive change'. As long as we feel we have made some shift in our state of mind, we have practised yoga. With this sūtra Patañjali clearly indicated the arena of change in yoga: it is our state of mind that is important and not necessarily our state of body (although obviously the two are often linked). According to this definition, stretching our hamstrings or strengthening our back, without positively changing our state of mind in the process, is not yoga.

3. YS 2.4, discussed more fully in Chapter 8.

4. These 5 are: misunderstanding (*avidyā*), confused sense of Self (*asmitā*), craving (*rāga*), repulsion (*dveṣa*) and fear (*abhiniveśa*). See Chapter 8 for further elaboration of *kleśa*.

Nirodha: The fundamental goal

Understanding the principle of *nirodha* is essential in order to fully appreciate the Yoga Sūtra. However, *nirodha* can be confusing for yoga students as it has a variety of different meanings within the text. The word comes from the Sanskrit root *rudh*, which means 'to obstruct', 'arrest', 'restrain' or 'cover'. This has led to many translations of YS 1.2 that are unhelpful. Fortunately, the principal commentator, Vyāsa, clarifies matters in his commentary to both sūtras 1.1 and 1.2. In YS 1.1, as we have noted, Vyāsa defines yoga as *samādhi*, a state of meditative absorption. He suggests that we can classify our state of mind into five categories, each of which has the potential for a type of *samādhi*. The first three can generate types of absorption that are obsessively active (*kṣipta*), dull and stuck (*mūḍha*), and clear but unstable (*vikṣipta*). These are not yogic states since they are not accompanied by both clarity and stability. The last two states, one-pointed (*ekāgra*) and 'arrested' (*niruddha* – a variation of the word *nirodha*) both have a high degree of clarity (*sattva guṇa*). Vyāsa further points out in his commentary to YS 1.2 that *both* of these are included in Patañjali's definition of yoga as *citta vṛtti nirodha*.

In the *ekāgra* state, the mind is focused in a chosen direction. All *vṛtti* reflect this direction, like the waves on the ocean moving together. Any *vṛtti* contrary to this direction are restrained and this is the essential meaning of *nirodha* here. Therefore, we could describe *nirodha* as 'channelling the activities of the mind towards the chosen area of focus'. The language used here needs to be understood carefully. There is definitely an act of will involved in maintaining the mind in a chosen direction, but brute force does not help! As any meditator will tell you, trying too hard is a surefire way to fail. It is necessary to '**take support**'. The first step is to create the right intention, and reapply our intention countless times as the mind wanders. However, this process of stabilising the mind is subtle and requires the attention to be 'held' by the object or direction of focus, so that the *nirodha* (or boundaries that determine what is active and what is restrained) is increasingly a *product of the process* rather than an imposition of will. The Yoga Sūtra provides us with more details about how this state may be cultivated in practice.

The final state of mind indicated by Vyāsa (*niruddha*) is one of deep meditation in which the mind has become very clear, subtle and quiet. *Niruddha* may arise from the practice of the previous state (*ekāgra*) with increasingly subtle levels of focus until all mental activity in the normal sense of the word has been temporarily suspended. From a practical point of view it is not something that we need to unduly concern ourselves with, as it is not something that can be easily 'practised',[5] and is well beyond the scope of this book. However, it is worth mentioning, if only to clear up a common mistake: students often conflate these two levels of *nirodha* and adopt as their guiding principle the aim to somehow 'stop their minds'. This is extremely unhelpful. The level of *nirodha* that we are seeking from our practice is *ekāgra*, where we are increasingly engaged, focused and absorbed.

Citta vṛtti nirodha offers the space to connect with ourselves

YS 1.3 tadā draṣṭuḥ sva-rūpe avasthānam

Then (in a state of yoga) there is space for what is profound in us to appear

Whereas the second sūtra gives us the fundamental definition of yoga, the third describes the fruit of achieving such a state. We shall explore the philosophical worldview of yoga in more depth in Chapter 7, but for now we simply need to appreciate that yoga proposes an enduring spiritual principle within all of us. This is separate to the material part of ourselves, which is seen as ever-changing, and

5. According to Vyāsa, it is possible to achieve *niruddha* by extensive practice of *ekāgra samādhi*, accompanied by the highest levels of *vairāgya*, but this is an extremely advanced practice.

thus subject to growth and eventual decay. This spiritual principle, our true Self, is given various names in the Yoga Sūtra but here is described as *draṣṭṛ*,[6] 'the one who sees'. It, rather than the mind, is the source of our consciousness or seeing.[7] Crucially, the mind is understood as material in nature because it is always in flux, as we all well know! This is extremely important to understand: according to yoga 'we' are not fundamentally our minds, but something beyond. The mind is seen as an instrument and possession of our true Self. It is the means *through* which we perceive and is also at the service of our true Self (just as a possession is owned and is at the service of its owner). Another name for this Self is *cit* ('pure awareness'), which is distinguished from the mind, *citta* ('that which relates to or is subservient to *cit*').

A very common theme in the Indian spiritual tradition is that although the mind and senses are at the service of the true Self, it requires great discipline and insight to maintain this relationship. In normal circumstances the mind and senses are frequently in control, driving us helplessly through a world of sensual experience and mental projection. Yoga is a journey to return the mind and the senses to their proper places (as servants or instruments of the Self). This restores our fundamental autonomy and freedom. Because the Self (*cit*) is unchanging, yoga is not about 'spiritual growth' – since spirit cannot and does not grow! Instead, it is about transforming what can be changed – our material nature, including our minds (*citta*), so that the Seer – our true Self – can manifest. According to this sūtra, when the mind becomes 'still' (or channelled appropriately), there is the space for the Seer to become more clearly present. This is reflected in the clarity of the mind. When the ripples on the surface of a pond settle we can see the bottom clearly. In a similar way when the mind becomes less disturbed and more stable, we have the possibility of seeing into the depths of our being.

We have already discussed the two primary levels of the state of *nirodha*. Here Patañjali is presenting the second

6. Embedded in the word *draṣṭuḥ*.

7. We could link *draṣṭṛ* to a more general awareness, but because it actually derives from the root *dṛś* meaning 'to see', we have defined it in these terms.

state, *niruddha*, and so this sūtra is concerned with very profound states of meditation that we may never achieve. However, what is remarkable about the Yoga Sūtra is that although many of its verses refer to deep states of meditative experience or esoteric philosophical ideas, many also relate to ordinary experiences. This is particularly true of this sūtra. At a very practical level, by creating a feeling of spaciousness and lightness, it is common to feel more intimately connected with ourselves, as even new yoga students will confirm. Such experiences, however fleeting, are valuable and should be cultivated. They are a catalyst for change that can begin to reorient our attitudes and values.

Traditional translations of the Yoga Sūtra describe the essential journey as inwards towards the ultimate realisation of the true Self. The third sūtra addresses the question: "When the mind is completely still in the highest level of *nirodha*, what is the state of the true Self, the Seer?" And the answer is: "Then the Seer stands in its own true form." Without any distortion from the *citta vṛtti*, the Seer is just as it is. Although very close to the mind and dependent on it for perception, here the Seer simply stands in its own true form – distinct from the mind, whose activities have temporarily ceased. This is part of the fundamental metaphysics of the Yoga Sūtra: it is how Patañjali sees the nature of the world and the nature of existence.

Although the 'highest level' of *nirodha* is elusive, we have all experienced moments when the mind's activities slow and settle – even if they do not cease entirely. These moments can leave us feeling deeply touched and reconnected to the most essential part of ourselves and to the greater process of Life, of which we are a part. As yoga teachers, we have observed this phenomenon of deep connection on many occasions: the atmosphere in the room changes, as if the space is being restructured in some way. Appearances can subtly change too so that people are no longer defined by their current state – young, old, woman, man, tired, tense, happy, sad. It is as if something timeless, beyond form, becomes present.

Cultivating space is another of our guiding principles. But what do we mean by 'space' and how do we cultivate it? Space here represents the quality of *sattva guṇa.*[8] *Sattva* is characterised by lightness and luminosity (connected to clarity of perception), and contrasted to principles of density and obscuration (*tamas*) on the one hand, and movement and stimulation (*rajas*) on the other. Thus, when we feel light (not heavy and dull) and clear (not preoccupied or over-stimulated), we have the space to connect to what is essentially most profound in us. The word 'essentially' here is significant – it indicates both what is *essence* (at the heart of our being), and what is *essential.* Without its presence, we would be without life, because in the yoga tradition it is the presence of the spiritual principle that animates our material nature with *prāṇa*, the energy of Life. Cultivating space is therefore a vital part of our yoga project and an important indicator that the practice has been effective.

It is common in yoga to focus on the various postures or techniques as if they have an intrinsic value in themselves, rather than being *the means* to refining ourselves. Focusing on the outcomes we are seeking gives a better indication of progress than, for example, mastery of a specific posture. Do we feel more spacious and therefore more connected to ourselves? This opens the door to innovation: if we have some ideas about what we are seeking then potentially anything that takes us in that direction could be considered yoga. The tension between tradition and innovation is a tricky path to negotiate. New schools of yoga spring up like mushrooms, each offering a new slant on the practice or a new fusion between traditional yoga and other ideas. But by using principles that have stood the test of time, we can characterise the yoga experience simply (e.g. 'the cultivation of space to deeply connect with ourselves') and thereby negotiate this minefield of 'too many possibilities'.[9]

8. See Chapter 7.

9. It's interesting that even in the 15th-century text *Haṭha Yoga Pradīpikā*, its author, Svātmārāma, bemoaned the state of yoga, saying that too many "wander in the darkness of conflicting doctrines" (HYP 1.3).

Identifying with our minds is an endless source of suffering

YS 1.4 vṛtti-sārūpyam itaratra

At other times, we identify with the contents of our minds

The last word of this sūtra, *itaratra,* means 'at other times' – when we are not in a state of *citta vṛttinirodha.* This is our usual state of mind: *vṛtti* constantly appear and there is little containment or direction of them. The tendency is then to identify with the activity and content of our minds – we get 'lost in thought' and our thoughts define who we think we are. When thoughts and feelings become very strong or entrenched, it seems that there is no separation between us and our minds. We are at the mercy of anxieties, neuroses and imagined ideas about how the world is, what it means, and our place within it. It is one thing to understand this intellectually, but another to stay true to that realisation at moments of high emotion. Our minds are very powerful and the *vṛtti* can easily become overwhelming.

This sūtra describes the spiritual Self (*cit, puruṣa or draṣṭṛ*) when the mind is active and not in a state of *nirodha.* The previous sūtra addressed its presence when the mind is still, and informed us that then the *draṣṭṛ* simply 'rests in its natural state'. Sūtra 1.4 says that at other times (when the *vṛtti* are active), its form (*sārūpyam* – where the 'it' is the *draṣṭṛ*) *is* the *vṛtti.* This leads us to a difficult metaphysical conundrum that needs some explaining. Fortunately, as with the previous sūtra, there is a very practical and understandable version that we will also present.

As we have stated, *puruṣa,*[10] the spiritual principle, is said to be unchanging and enduring, in contrast to the materiality of the world around us, our bodies, and, most importantly, our minds. If *puruṣa* is unchanging then it must be the same regardless of whether the *citta vṛtti* are active or subdued in the state of *nirodha.* However, sūtra 1.3 tells us that in *nirodha* the *puruṣa* simply 'rests in its own form',

10. Although we have previously referred to *draṣṭṛ, puruṣa* is a more common term.

and in sūtra 1.4 we understand its form is the *vṛtti*. We have an apparent contradiction: something that is unchanging and in its true form, cannot, by definition, become other than that. Its form cannot suddenly become that of the *vṛtti*. This has led to some differences of opinion even among traditional commentators, but the answer seems both straightforward and yet raises more questions that are not ever fully answered. In most philosophical systems and scientific theories that attempt to explain the complexities of reality using conceptual language, there usually comes a point where the logic breaks down and either we are left with an essential mystery, or the system is accepted as an approximation of the reality that it describes.

Vyāsa provides an explanation. During normal consciousness, although the *puruṣa* does not change, it appears as if it changes its form with the *vṛtti*. In fact, because all we *can* be aware of are the *vṛtti*, we can do little else but assume that they reflect who we truly are, since we do not experience anything else. In other words, all experience is in the mind. Even when we observe our minds in meditation, noticing the arising and passing of thoughts and feelings, the noticing itself is nothing other than another *vṛtti*, another perception in the mind. The mind is all we have in terms of generating experience no matter how subtle it may become.

Does this mean we are doomed, in an endless spiral of *vṛtti* with no escape from the matrix of our minds? Not exactly: even insights arising in our own mind, about the nature of other *vritti* in the same mind (as when observing our thoughts and feelings), give us insight into the way our mind works. This enables us to identify with it less completely. Insight into the way things are has the possibility of changing what actually happens. In truth, it is actually the mind that adopts the form of the *vṛtti*, not the *puruṣa*, and it is the continuity of this experience in the mind that gives rise to our conventional sense of identity. So, we might interpret YS 1.4 as stating that 'at other times, when the mind is active, the mind assumes the form of thoughts, feelings, memories and perceptions that are arising and, because we fundamentally misunderstand the relationship between our true Self and the mind, we identify with that'. In short, we identify with the projections of our own mind.

Let us return to our working definition of YS 1.4 above, "at other times, we tend to identify with the contents of our minds". This is the bottom line, even if the metaphysics seems impenetrable. The identification with the *citta vṛtti* is problematic because they can easily become overwhelming or self-perpetuating, and lead to experiences of suffering and distress. Much of our mental content is, in fact, a projection or distortion of the reality of ourselves and the world around us, and our anxieties about the future or memories of the past can prevent us from being really present. So, who on earth would want a mind, if it is the cause of so much distortion and distress?

The role of the mind and the *citta vṛtti* in causing suffering is only half the story. Indian philosophy is sometimes accused of being overly negative, but this is only because it focuses on the causes of suffering and how to address them. We should also appreciate what a remarkable instrument the mind is. Without it we would have no experience, no faculties of perception, no positive human qualities such as love and compassion, and no means to navigate life's journey. When it is clear and focused, and the internal projections and distortions of reality are minimised, it enables acute perception, reasoning and creativity. These qualities free us from the tyrannies of habit, dullness and agitation. We will explore such states of clarity in Chapter 15 where the process of meditation and the potential results are discussed in more detail.

Sādhana: *Nirodha* is both method and goal

The definition of yoga as *citta vṛtti nirodha* defines the goal of the practice: to achieve a state of *nirodha*. However, it also defines the method. It is common in the Yoga Sūtra for definitions of states also to give us the principles to reach those states. For example, āsana is defined by the qualities of stability (*sthira)* and comfort (*sukha*). This gives us a clue to its methodology: the active cultivation of *sthira* and *sukha.*[11] In a similar way, employing *nirodha* as method, is the means to cultivate the goal.

Nirodha as method is the process of focusing, channelling and containing. The yoga tradition has always acknowledged and worked with the relationship between body, breath and mind. We can apply the principles of *nirodha* to these three domains, so we can work with *kāya nirodha* (*nirodha* of the body), *prāṇa nirodha*, (*nirodha* of the breath or vital energy) and *citta vṛtti nirodha*, (*nirodha* of the mind). These are interdependent: *nirodha* of the body and breath support *nirodha* of the mind.

In Chapter 1, we discussed an important aspect of *kāya nirodha*: 'learning to be still'. Being still is a literal *nirodha* of the body and provides an opportunity for the energy of the system to settle. It also provides a stable backdrop to cultivating our inner awareness. But the scope of *kāya nirodha* is far wider within our āsana practice. *Nirodha* as channelling or containing also applies to the dynamic aspects of the practice, i.e. how we move into and out of āsana. When working dynamically we cultivate smooth, even movements within a prescribed set of steps (*vinyāsa krama*).[12] The form of the movement into and out of an āsana is prescribed; it is not random and should not be embellished with either artistic flourishes or unconscious twitches. It is channelled and contained within the *vinyāsa krama*. There is a simple and direct quality in our movement.

Dynamic work in āsana and in āsana sequences,[13] where we link several postures together in a flow, can be very

11. See Chapter 9.

12. See Chapter 3.

13. See Chapter 7.

engaging. We need to add a note of caution here, however. Flowing sequences can be hypnotic, so we need to be vigilant to remain present. It is easy to lose oneself within flowing sequences, as if switching off and trancing out when you dance. This can give some relief from the constant dialogue in the mind, but is contrary to the principle in yoga of being present with focus and clarity (the characteristics of *sattva guṇa*). Trancelike states may be dominated by the dull absorption typical of *tamas* or the energetic passion of *rajas*. Performed with care and attention, sequences can be great for engaging our energy when we need to wake the body up, or need somewhere to channel a build-up of energy in the body – as long as they encourage us to stay present rather than switch off.

Static āsana are a literal *nirodha* of the body in that they further contain the body. Generally, there is a progression from more movement towards more stillness, both over the course of a single practice and as a development of practice over the longer term. Breath work is most intensely focused in static postures and, consequently, they provide the ideal arena for directing the mind. *Kāya nirodha* finds its ultimate expression in the ability to sit for a long time without disturbance from the body, so that we can engage in static practices such as prāṇāyāma and meditation.

Prāṇa nirodha, channelling and containing the movement of the breath, uses similar principles. Because there is movement during inhalation and exhalation, they are like the dynamic aspect of āsana. In prāṇāyāma, or indeed in the way that we breathe in āsana, the first step is to regulate the inhalation and exhalation to make the breath long, smooth and even. This is the channelling aspect of *nirodha* applied to the breath. The breath is linked to movement in dynamic āsana and directed more precisely in static āsana. In prāṇāyāma, the flow of the breath is then channelled and directed further by the posture, which is specifically structured for this purpose.

Although *prāṇa* can sometimes be understood to mean the breath, it also refers to the vital energy which underpins all our movement – physical, breathing or even activity in the mind. Yoga acknowledges the intimate relationship between our breath and *prāṇa* so that in using the term *prāṇa* we are often referring to both the breath and the vital energy to which it is so intimately linked. Working with the breath directly influences our *prāṇa* and changes in the state of our *prāṇa* are reflected in the breath. The final link in the chain is the mind (*citta*). As a famous verse from the *Haṭha Yoga Pradīpikā* states, 'When *prāṇa* moves, the mind moves; when *prāṇa* is still, the mind is still' (HYP 2.2). So working with the breath is a means to directly influence our *prāṇa* and therefore our mind. Simply stand in *samasthiti*, take a few long smooth breaths in *ujjāyī*,[14] and the mind feels calmer; the effect is very direct. New students can be surprised when they first discover *ujjāyī*. Taking long, smooth, regulated breaths they often immediately experience a lighter, more spacious feeling. Krishnamacharya said, "Haṭha Yoga **is** prāṇāyāma," and here we might go further: Haṭha Yoga is *prāṇa nirodha* and it directly creates the conditions for *citta vṛtti nirodha*.

'Breath work is most intensely focused in static postures and, consequently, they provide the ideal arena for directing the mind.'

Pausing at the end of the inhale or exhale (*kumbhaka)* is like static āsana in that it reflects the principle of *nirodha* as absolute containment or cessation most directly. Although requiring care in its application, the principle of *kumbhaka* (where the breath is suspended or paused in āsana and prāṇāyāma), opens up a space for the most profound experiences of stillness. Because of the direct link between breath, *prāṇa* and *citta*, *kumbhaka* can cultivate profound moments of *citta vṛtti nirodha* directly. This has been explored to its limits within the Haṭha Yoga tradition.[15]

In practice, *kāya nirodha* and *prāṇa nirodha* support *citta vṛtti nirodha,* and many of the practical elements of the

14. See Chapter 9.

15. See Chapter 10.

methodology in this approach can be understood in terms of the principle of *nirodha* – it is like a master key that explains why we practise the way we do. However, *citta vṛtti nirodha* is also an element that must be brought directly into the practice and not just considered as a consequence of the other levels.

This requires us to focus our minds, and engage deeply and consistently with the practice. Often it is maintaining our focus that is the greatest challenge. A number of elements in the practice are direct supports for our attention, such as the feeling of *ujjāyī* in the throat and many of the postural cues that encourage us to pay close attention to our bodies during āsana. However, we need to be active and diligent in making the effort to link and stay with them. *Bhāvana*[16] are specific elements to focus on. They are designed to engage the mind by cultivating a feeling or image, thereby channelling and directing the *vṛtti*. The most effective *bhāvana* draw us into subtle and deep levels of focused experience.

Nirodha is therefore the underlying principle of all yoga practice. When you next step onto the mat, consider all the elements of the practice that encourage *nirodha* at the three levels of body, breath and mind. In the final analysis, yoga is *citta vṛtti nirodha*, so don't just be a passenger: make a conscious intention and effort to focus and link with all the supportive elements of the practice, and seek to maintain this throughout. This can be demanding irrespective of the physical effort of performing difficult postures and precisely why the simplest of practices can produce the most profound results if approached with the right attitude. This is real yoga.

16. See Chapter 16.

Chapter 3

तस्य भूमिषु विनियोगः ।

Starting from Where You Are

YS 3.6 tasya bhūmiṣu viniyogaḥ

According to the level and circumstances of the student, thus the application

This sūtra is the only place in the whole text where the word *viniyoga* is used. *Viniyoga* simply means 'application' and, in this sense, it is not specifically connected with yoga at all (it is not '*vini-Yoga*' – a '*vini*' approach to yoga). The prefix *vi* is short for *viśeṣa*, which means 'specific and distinct'; the body of the word is *niyoga,* meaning 'application'. We would be more correct, therefore, to talk about the *viniyoga* of yoga – the specific application of yoga.

According to this sūtra, only when a step has been firmly established (*bhūmiṣu*) should one progress to the next level. The size and direction of each step is dependent on the practitioner; there is no universal standard. Although this sūtra comes in Chapter 3 of the Yoga Sūtra and specifically refers to the practice of meditation, its scope is much wider: it suggests we apply the practices and techniques of yoga while respecting the capacity, interest, and circumstances of the student.

Viniyoga: Individual and group classes

The individual application of yoga is an essential principle that is easily forgotten in the modern yoga scene with its multitude of styles, celebrities and body culture. It runs counter to the idea of yoga as an idealised practice, form or sequence to which all students aspire. Desikachar, like his father Krishnamacharya, was adamant that yoga should serve the student and be tailored to individual needs. Desikachar did not teach a 'style' of yoga, because each person is different. It was for this reason that he became unhappy with calling his approach to yoga 'Viniyoga' – it sounds too much like a style or a brand. He described how he was never entirely happy with the name 'Viniyoga', but adopted it while at a yoga conference in Zinal, Switzerland in the early 1980s where he was asked what his approach was called. The story is that he consulted his father, and Krishnamacharya suggested 'Viniyoga' as it encapsulated something of the idea of individualised application. But unfortunately, by 'branding' it thus, we are in danger of reducing an approach to a style, which everybody practises in the same way, and so a sort of rigid orthodoxy begins to develop.

While we often associate practising yoga with going to a yoga class or yoga centre, Desikachar emphasised yoga as a personal discipline, ideally to be practised alone in our own environment. The German yoga scholar Georg Feuerstein once described yoga as "what you do when no one else is looking". The practice is personal and it creates space to cultivate our relationship with ourselves. The principle of *viniyoga* as 'skilful application' cannot be overemphasised. However, it begs the question: what is an appropriate practice for me? The ideal answer to this is to find someone who specialises in designing and teaching individual practices. Take some time to find a teacher to whom you can relate. The relationship between student and teacher has always been considered fundamental to our progress in yoga, and Desikachar considered the individual teaching of yoga to be paramount.

Individual and group classes are rather different in their intention. Individual classes allow the student to develop a more profound relationship with the teacher, and often, in individual classes, many aspects of the student's life can be aired and discussed. For us, both as teachers and as students, we feel privileged to have had such profound connections with fellow travellers in one-to-one classes. An individual class is geared to developing and sustaining a home practice, and there is space for direct feedback on one's practice so that refinements and adjustments can be made in greater detail than that afforded in the average group class.

Traditional individual classes are primarily concerned with home practice, while students in a group class often only practise during that session. For the student, it can often be difficult to know how to translate what is done in a group class into an effective and appropriate home practice. Undoubtedly the group class can be a supportive and nurturing setting in which to practise and an opportunity to engage in a shared pursuit with a group of like-minded people. Often people move on from the group class to individual lessons, or even supplement group lessons with individual ones. Many of our group-class students say that the class is the best part of their week – an oasis of calm within the maelstrom of life. Although group classes are general by their very nature, a good teacher should be able to modify practices and postures to accommodate a range of abilities. However, do take time to find a class that suits you: they are often different in what they emphasise, and how physically demanding they are.

Adapting our practice

Although we will be presenting a number of postures, techniques and practice principles in this book, it is important to remember that they need to be approached within your own limits. It has never been intended for everyone to practise everything. Even though the yoga tradition has explored the extreme limits of human possibility in working with the body, the breath and the mind, much of this is not relevant or even possible for most people. However, it is possible to achieve profound results with the simplest of practices skilfully chosen and practised with care. As long as we can still breathe, we can practise yoga – it does not necessarily mean we all need to stand on our heads! Equally, what is appropriate for us to practise at twenty-five may not be possible or even desirable in our seventies. As we get older, mature and change, our practice will need to adapt. Yoga is about meeting change creatively. At some point, inevitably, our physical abilities will begin to diminish, but this does not mean our yoga practice must necessarily decline. It is worth remembering that yoga is concerned with the depth of our experience and not necessarily our physical capacity.

Four stages of life: *brahmacarya*, *gṛhastha*, *vanaprastha* and *saṃnyāsa*

As we grow older, our priorities, interests and possibilities change. Although there is no absolute standard progression to the way in which we grow, Vedic culture divided the progression into four parts (or *āśrama*):

- *brahmacarya* – youth
- *gṛhastha* – householder
- *vanaprastha* – retired
- *saṃnyāsa* – renunciate

For youngsters, with plenty of energy and potential for growth, the Ancients emphasised a focus on study and the cultivation of helpful habits. This stage, *brahmacarya* (which is often translated as sexual abstinence), is about defining and maintaining our priorities in life. Rather than dissipate our considerable energies and potentials, the emphasis here is on developing the self-discipline to support us as we meet life's various challenges.

As we get older, we commonly partner up and many of us have children. Of course there are many joys during this time, but we also become more involved with our responsibilities – caring for our children, for our aging parents, providing an income and contributing to society. In many ways, it is a pivotal time and demands are made on us from above, below, sideways, inside and out! Ideally, the energy and focus developed during our *brahmacarya* years will help us to navigate the challenges of the years of *gṛhastha* ('grasped by, or occupied with, the household').

The next stage of life is called *vanaprastha* – literally 'establishing oneself in the forest'. It is most close to our retirement phase; it may involve downsizing; it certainly should be a reprioritising of one's interior journey, and a letting go of the reins. As our work in the external world becomes less important, our spiritual work becomes more so. This is a time to move towards deep meditation; it is a time for reflection and letting be.

The final stage, *saṃnyāsa,* is something of an anomaly because it is not necessarily age-specific. This is complete renunciation and the word is used for spiritual mendicants: those who have given up their worldly lives to devote themselves to spiritual pursuits at whatever stage of life. It involves deep reflection, study and practice, and here the central concern is liberation (*mokṣa*). It is not necessarily a stage that we will all go through, and there are those who become *saṃnyāsins* very early in their lives (although how appropriate this is will surely vary).

We can link these stages of life, somewhat poetically, to the phases of the breath (which, too, are cyclical):

- *brahmacarya* with the inhalation (*pūraka*): opening to the world.
- *gṛhastha* with the pause after the inhalation (*antar kumbhaka*): staying with the world.
- *vanaprastha* with the exhalation (*recaka*): releasing to the world.

- *saṃnyāsa* with the pause after the exhalation (*bāhya kumbhaka*): surrendering of the world.

Three approaches to practice: *sṛṣṭikrama, sthitikrama* and *layakrama*

There is some debate about the authenticity of Nāthamuni's text on yoga called *Yoga Rahasya* ('The Secret of Yoga'). Nāthamuni, a revered ninth-century sage from Southern India, and also one of Krishnamacharya's ancestors, is said to have appeared to the sixteen-year-old Krishnamacharya in a dream and dictated the lost text, *Yoga Rahasya*, which Krishnamacharya then committed to memory. Although a powerful romantic story, Desikachar himself stated:

> "My father never acknowledged that he discovered anything even when I have seen that it was he who discovered [*sic*]. He has discovered postures but he would say that it was his teacher who taught him. Rarely has he said that it was his 'original' work...I tend to think that the Nāthamuni's *Yogarahasya [sic]* that he taught us is quite likely to be a combination of his own commentary and the lessons he received..."[1]

The text certainly contains many important principles which were hallmarks of both Krishnamacharya and Desikachar's teachings; indeed Chapter 5 is called *Viniyogādhyāyaḥ* – in which Nāthamuni presents three approaches to yoga practice:

- *sṛṣṭikrama* (also known as *vṛddhi*) – focus on growth
- *sthitikrama* – focus on stability
- *layakrama* (also known as *antar*) – focus on dissolution

The first of these, *sṛṣṭikrama,* is concerned with strengthening and challenging the developing body. Here, the emphasis is on the cultivation of āsana, on exploring the limits of possibilities and thereby gaining good physical and mental health, as well as creating a foundation of good habits and a certain steadiness and discipline. This practice is to be

1. Extract from an interview with TKV Desikachar in *Darśanam 1*, no 1, Feb 1991. Krishnamacharya Yoga Mandiram.

undertaken during the *brahmacarya* years when we are still growing; it becomes the bedrock for the rest of our lives. Although prāṇāyāma and meditative practices are introduced and practised, they are less important than āsana.

Sthitikrama, as its name implies, is concerned with stability and is the approach to yoga for those in the *gṛhastha* stage of life. During this time, the demands of family life can unsettle us, and easily knock us off balance. In this phase, it may be difficult to devote large amounts of time to one's study and practice of yoga and the priority here is to maintain good physical and psychological health. Krishnamacharya felt that the priority during this time is prāṇāyāma, although obviously āsana has an extremely important role to play in helping to keep our bodies strong and flexible. More than anything else, prāṇāyāma is the practice for mental stability and resilience.

Finally, *layakrama* is primarily concerned with the practice of meditation, of reflection and study. *Layakrama* is important for those in the *vanaprastha* and *saṃnyāsa* stages, where there is more reviewing of life, a withdrawal from the maelstrom of jobs and family responsibilities and the beginnings of preparation for death. Here, *vairāgya*[2] is an important aspect of practice as we mature into a new stage of life.

Three aims in practice: *śikṣaṇa krama*, *rakṣaṇa krama* and *cikitsā krama*

There will be times in our lives when we are able to devote considerable energy and enthusiasm to developing something new in our yoga practice and thereby push our boundaries. But there will be other times when the possibilities for yoga practice are more limited, perhaps due to lack of time or to other circumstances. Young or old, we can also experience illness at any age or stage of our lives; sometimes it will be short-lived and at others it may be life-

2. *Vairāgya* is one of the two fundamental principles of Patañjali's system. It is often translated as 'non-attachment' but for a more detailed discussion see Chapter 5.

changing and permanent. Importantly, our practice need not stay the same throughout such fluctuations; indeed, the purpose of the 'viniyoga of yoga' is to refine our approach so that it most appropriately supports our current life circumstances.

Krishnamacharya and Desikachar skilfully used three broad categories to address the types of practice that we might undertake at different times. It is extremely helpful to understand these classifications because they open up the possibilities of yoga practice to anybody and they provide some guiding principles for our direction and purpose. They are:

- *śikṣaṇa krama* – yoga practice for spiritual transformation, without compromise
- *rakṣaṇa krama* – yoga practice which maintains our energy and helps to protect us
- *cikitsā krama* – yoga practice as therapy

These three principles can be applied in any arena, whether it is āsana, prāṇāyāma or meditation. A *śikṣaṇa* practice implies intensity; techniques are taught and then practised without modifications. In order to work in such a way, there should be no limiting factors and no reason to dilute the intensity of the practice. The sort of āsana practice that Krishnamacharya taught to Patabhi Jois[3] and BKS Iyengar[4] in the 1930s was *śikṣaṇa*. They were young men who could take on very strong physical practices, appropriate to the *sṛṣṭikrama* stage of life. This sort of āsana practice can readily be part of a *viniyoga* practice but it is unwise to attempt strong and uncompromised āsana if your physical or energetic systems are unable to maintain such a practice, lest you injure yourself or simply find the practice unsustainable. We could also apply the principle of *śikṣaṇa krama* to prāṇāyāma. Here we would need to be able to sit very easily on the floor in *padmāsana* or similar and stay there for a minimum of fifteen minutes while maintaining a long and slow breath.

Rakṣaṇa is the act of protecting, and a *rakṣaṇa krama*

3. Patabhi Jois (1915–2009), one of Krishnamacharya's students from Mysore was the guru of the Ashtanga Vinyasa (sic) Krama school of yoga, which has become one of the most popular approaches to āsana. It is an intensely aerobic system with six levels, each progressively more demanding. Very few have mastered sequences beyond Level 3.

4. BKS Iyengar (1918–2014), another of Krishnamacharya's students from Mysore and also his brother-in-law, is probably the most famous yoga teacher in the West. His approach to refining āsana demanded great perseverance and commitment from students and although he modified his approach in later life, he was known for his strictness, his intensity and his lack of compromise.

practice is one that is sustainable and supports us. It helps to protect us physically, mentally and psychologically. The effects of overly sedentary modern lifestyles caused by (and causing) lack of movement and poor posture can be countered by a regular *rakṣaṇa krama* practice. This is about the long-term care of our joints, our backs, our breath and our mental health. It is a sort of 'top up' which helps to mitigate the effects of the 'energy expenditure' that modern lifestyles require. For most people, and certainly for most people in the *gṛhastha* stage of life, *rakṣaṇa krama* is the most appropriate practice as we are far less likely to injure ourselves, or to find the commitment to maintain a *śikṣaṇa* practice.

Finally, yoga can be extremely effective as a therapy and then it is called *cikitsā krama*. Here the goal is to recover our health as best we can. We may have hurt our back temporarily, or we may have a chronic condition which we need to take care of for the rest of our lives. In such cases, attempting *śikṣaṇa* or even sometimes *rakṣana* practices may result in further injury or depletion. *Cikitsā krama* practices are usually characterised by being very accessible, gentle and not too long. Techniques are modified appropriately and the emphasis is on a daily practice to help us deal with the condition and, hopefully, to recover and perhaps take on a more intense or demanding practice when we are able.

In discussing these concepts, yoga teacher Paul Harvey[5] often used a particularly effective analogy which he called "the energetic bank balance". He described *śikṣaṇa* practice as appropriate when we have "money in the bank" – we are able to spend, invest and really do something with our assets. *Rakṣana* practice helps us to keep solvent, topping up our energetic bank balance that we deplete in the course of our daily lives. Finally, *cikitsā krama* is necessary when we are overdrawn and need to bring ourselves back into the black, so to speak, and thereby to return to optimum health.

5. Personal communication.

Two types of practice: *laṅghana kriyā* and *bṛṃhaṇa kriyā*

As well as being an extremely skilled practitioner of yoga and a renowned scholar of traditional Vedic philosophy, Krishnamacharya was also highly trained in āyurveda and he used many concepts from āyurveda in his application of yoga. The concepts of *laṅghana kriyā* and *bṛṃhaṇa kriyā* come directly from āyurveda where they are used to describe two different types of therapy. *Laṅghana kriyā* are treatments aimed at reducing body tissue and/or impurities in the system where there is excess; such treatments include sweating, fasting and purging. The aim of *laṅghana kriyā* is *laghu* – lightness. In contrast, *bṛṃhaṇa kriyā,* derived from the root *bṛh* meaning to expand, is about increasing tissue. Its techniques include sleeping, oiling and eating to gain weight.

Krishnamacharya used the same terms when he applied them to yoga techniques, but their effects are somewhat different. *Laṅghana kriyā* techniques in yoga focus on the exhalation and their primary area of activity is below the diaphragm in the abdomen. They quite literally make the body lighter, because the exhalation is linked to expulsion and reduction. *Laṅghana* āsana include any which are entered into with an exhalation: forward bends, which compress the abdomen, are the classic *laṅghana* postures. Their effect is to reduce. We can subdivide *laṅghana kriyā* into two further categories: calming and soothing practices (*śamana*), and strong energetic purification (*śodhana*). The former, focusing on exhalations and gentle forward bends, help lessen mental agitation and stimulation and soothe the system (e.g. *apanāsana,* fig 3.1).

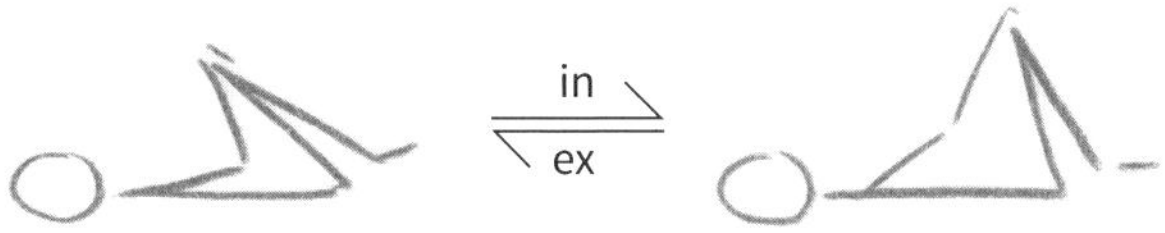

fig 3.1

The latter offers more intense practices which include strong compression in the abdomen and perhaps lengthy exhalations and *bāhya kumbhaka*[6] (e.g. *jānu śīrṣāsana*, fig 3.2, and *paścimatānāsana*, fig 3.3). These practices also have a *laṅghana* effect, but are more about energetic purification (*śodhana*) than simple soothing.

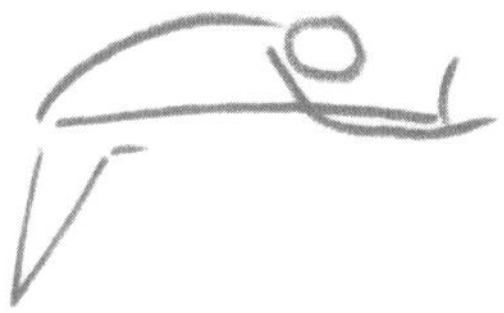

fig 3.2

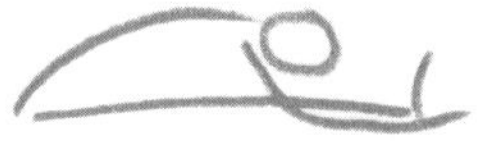

fig 3.3

Whilst *laṅghana* techniques either reduce mental agitation or excess tissue and toxicity in the body, *bṛṃhaṇa kriyā* primarily focus on the inhalation and usually have something of a stimulating effect. The sternum lifts, the chest expands and the spine arches backward. The most common *bṛṃhaṇa* āsana are backward bends such as *vīrabhadrāsana* (fig 3.4) and *bhujaṅgāsana* (fig 3.5).

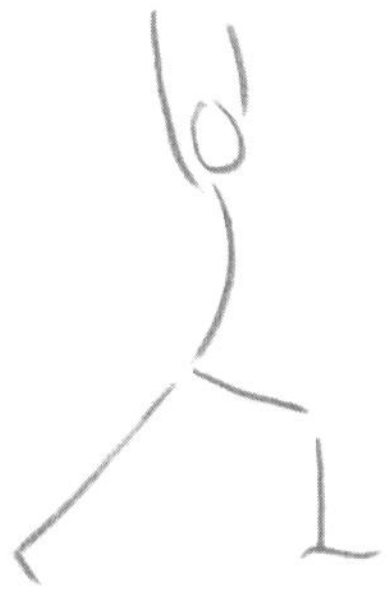

fig 3.4

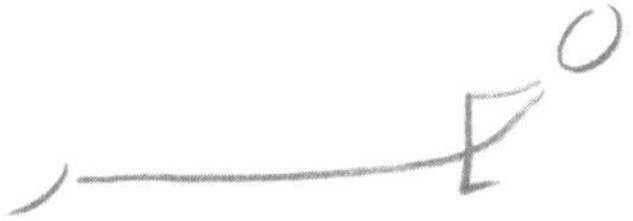

fig 3.5

Although these techniques usually have something of an uplifting and stimulating effect, if one is already tired, a strong *bṛṃhaṇa* practice can leave one feeling exhausted.

Twists have elements of both compression (in the abdomen) and also expansion (in the chest – particularly on one side). Consequently, they are classified as *laṅghana*

6. Pause at the end of the exhalation. See Chapter 10 for detailed discussion.

miśra (mixed). Their primary action is that of reduction and exhalation, but because of the lengthening of the spine and expansion of the chest, they also have elements of *bṛṃhaṇa kriyā*. Twists usually have quite a stimulating effect; there is something purifying about their action which may leave us feeling lighter and therefore more energetic. Examples include *parivṛtti trikonāsana* (fig 3.6) and *ardha matsyendrāsana* (fig 3.7).

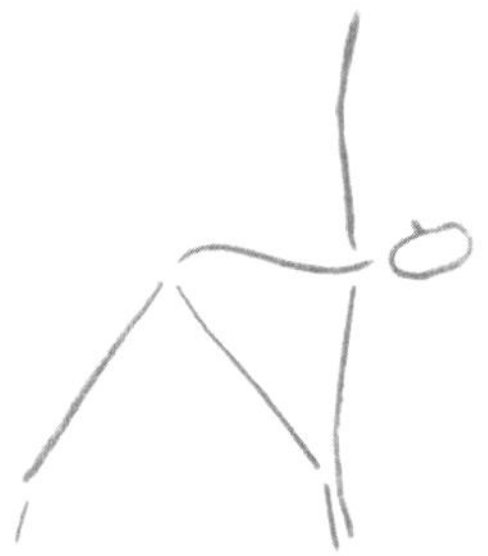

fig 3.6

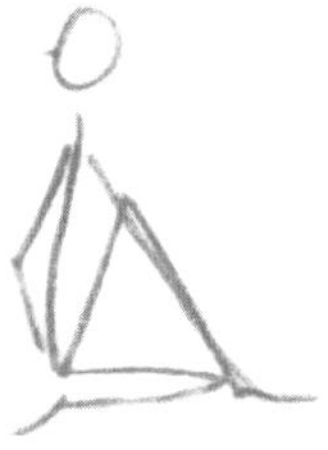

fig 3.7

Four purposes to life: *puruṣārtha*

The ancient Seers of India (the *ṛṣis*) outlined four purposes to life, irrespective of who we are. They appreciated that different people have different capacities and interests, and while paths may differ, the ultimate goals remain the same for everyone. The four purposes (*puruṣārtha*) are:

- *dharma* – doing that which supports us and others; playing our part appropriately
- *artha* – the means by which we make a living
- *kāma* – sensual enjoyment, pleasure
- *mokṣa* – liberation

These four elements should work harmoniously with each other. Ideally, *dharma* and *mokṣa* function like the banks of a river, directing the flow *of artha* and *kāma*. In other words, making a living and finding pleasure are tempered and contextualised by our commitment to doing the right thing and also to pursuing our spiritual goals.

Unfortunately, all too easily the roles are reversed: *artha* and *kāma* become the banks and the flow of *dharma* and *mokṣa* is defined by the pursuit of pleasure and wealth. Thus fulfilling our responsibilities becomes a chore which restricts our pleasure, and spirituality becomes a fashion accessory for our lifestyles. When our senses override our wisdom and we are pulled towards their gratification, our ability to stand back and reflect on what is most important is severely compromised.

Not only did the *ṛṣis* see people as having different priorities in relationship to their goals, they also acknowledged that everyone has different capacities, interests and possibilities. What is our *dharma*? What is appropriate work? What does freedom mean and how can we responsibly engage with money and wealth? Honest self-reflection is required.

Sādhana: *Vinyāsa krama*

> "We start our practice where we are and look towards a certain goal. Then we choose the steps that will lead us toward realizing that goal and will then gradually bring us back into our everyday life. But our daily practice does not return us to the exact place we started. The practice has changed us."
>
> TKV Desikachar, *Heart of Yoga*[7]

It is essential to first understand the concept of *vinyāsa krama*, and then to apply it. The word *nyāsa* (embedded here in '*vinyāsa*') means 'to place'; and here, the prefix '*vi*' is an abbreviation of the word *viśeṣa,* meaning 'special' or 'distinct'.[8] So *vinyāsa* means a 'special, specific or intelligent placing'. The second word, *krama*, means 'step'. Thus *vinyāsa krama* is the intelligent ordering of a number of steps that lead us to a particular goal. There may be a number of different routes to climb a mountain, but the experience

7. TKV Desikachar, *Heart of Yoga: Developing a Personal Practice* Inner Traditions, 1999, p. 26.

8. Here the prefix is the same as in *vi-niyoga*. However, in different contexts *vi* can mean 'opposite to'

of standing at the summit will be in part defined by our ascent. Gandhi once stated that the means cannot justify the end, because the means *are* the end. How we create an experience defines that experience; *vinyāsa krama* is simply the sequence of steps that we take to create an experience.

Vinyāsa krama of posture

There are a number of tools that help us towards the goal of stability and ease in posture (*sthirasukham āsanam*).[9] One of the most important of these is *vinyāsa krama*. If you come into a yoga posture with no awareness, with scant attention to the breath, or with an attitude of grasping, you will limit the possibility of stability (*sthira*) and comfort (*sukha*). To really cultivate the play of *sthira* and *sukha* in a posture, we must be involved and sensitive to the subtle nuances of the breath and body as they dance together. This involvement and sensitivity needs to be present during the whole posture – that is: how we enter, how we stay, and how we leave and complete the posture.

Every posture has a starting point, a position of neutrality to which we can return on completion of the posture. We call these 'link postures'. For any of the standing poses, the starting point is *samasthiti* – standing with attention (fig 3.8).

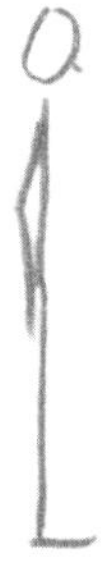

fig 3.8

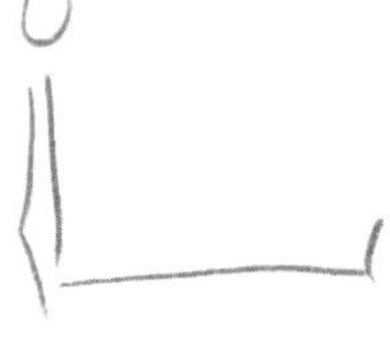

fig 3.9

For seated poses, the link posture is *daṇḍāsana* (fig 3.9), sitting upright with the legs straight out in front.

9. For a detailed explanation of YS 2.46 (*sthirasukham āsanam*) see Chapter 9.

From these positions, we synchronise our breath with various movements of the limbs and the trunk in order to come to the final posture. This may take one or more breaths. And, while there will be a 'standard' way of moving in and out of the posture (*śikṣaṇa* or 'uncompromised' form), there can also be many alternative *vinyāsa krama* which may modify our experience to emphasise a particular aspect of the pose. Thus, for example, the standard *vinyāsa* into *dvi pāda pīṭham* involves starting with bent legs and lifting the hips on an inhalation (fig 3.10):

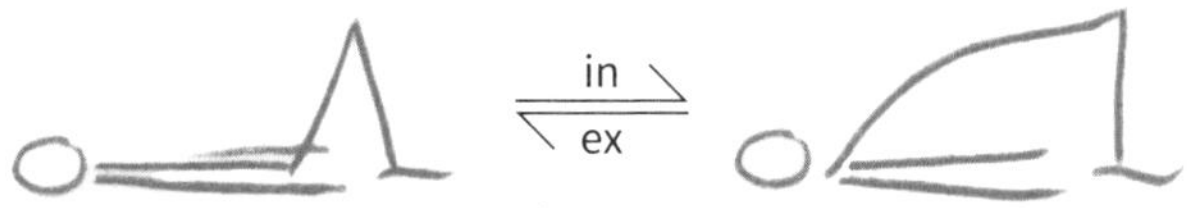

fig 3.10

For some, however, the effort to come into the posture with a *śikṣaṇa* approach may not cultivate either *sthira or sukha*. Perhaps entering *dvi pāda pīṭham* in this way pinches the back, or causes strain – there may be too much *sthira* which can compromise the feeling of *sukha*. So we need to consider alternative, softer ways of approaching the form. We could, for example, enter the posture on an exhale, remain as we inhale, and descend on the exhale (fig 3.11).

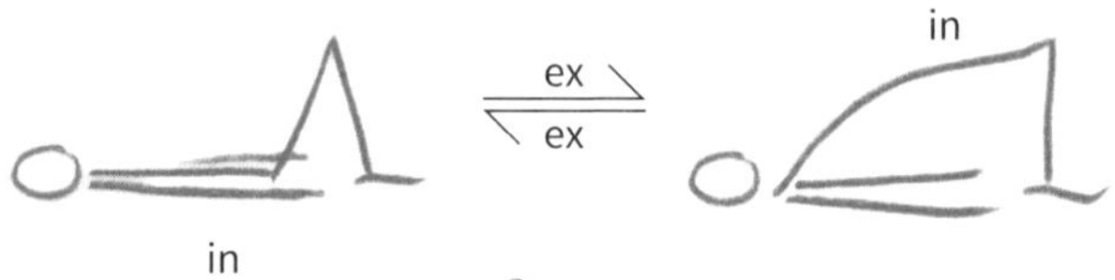

fig 3.11

For some, perhaps their familiarity with the form compromises attention. It is easy to switch off to what we are very used to and so simple variations can maintain our interest, revitalising the relationship between *sthira* and *sukha*. The standard *vinyāsa* for entering the warrior posture is this (fig 3.12):

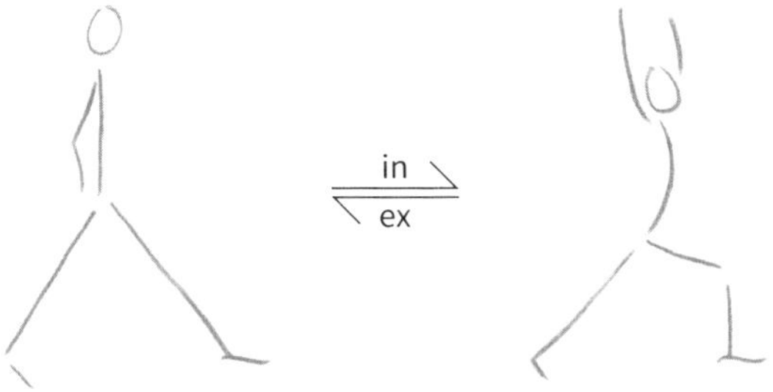

fig 3.12

To make a more challenging *vinyāsa*, we could create a sequence such as in fig 3.13.

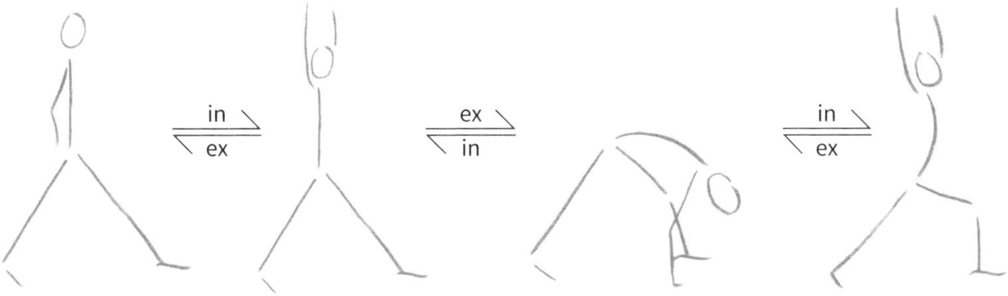

fig 3.13

An understanding of the *śikṣaṇa vinyāsa krama* of a posture, and how this may be varied and modified, is essential to creative involvement with āsana.

Vinyāsa krama of practice

Just as a single posture has a number of steps, so too can we apply the concept of *vinyāsa krama* to a whole practice. It is important to emphasise here that we are talking about principles rather than rules. If we understand the principles, we can change them as appropriate. Without such an understanding, we may produce ragged, ill-conceived practices which can lead to inefficiency, dissipation and, worse, to actual harm. Injuries can occur when there is insufficient or inappropriate preparation or counterposture in āsana, and the skilful design of practices is essential to refining our safe progress in yoga.

By ordering the groups of postures, we can come up with a simple acronym that is useful as our starting point: SKLIBS. We begin with standing postures (S), then take kneeling (K), lying (L), inverted (I), (prone) backward bends (B), and finally seated postures (S). Of course, in practice we may not actually perform postures from all of these groups, but this ordering has an internal consistency and logic that makes it a good default.

Standing postures

Standing postures all start from *samasthiti*. By starting with standing postures, we begin in a position closest to normal life. We usually work with eyes open in standing postures (which are generally less meditative), forming a bridge or gateway into the deeper and more introspective work that comes later. Keeping the eyes open is also helpful for balance. Because the spine and hips are free in space, standing postures also offer us the largest range of movement; there is greater possibility of free movement in a standing forward bend or twist than in their seated equivalents. This freedom allows us to cultivate and refine the breath, to develop flexibility and to 'get things moving'; they are a preparation for more challenging static postures later in the practice. In Sanskrit, we talk of *prāṇa calana*, the circulation of energy, and standing postures are ideal for this. These could include *pārśva uttānāsana* (fig 3.14), *parivṛtti trikonāsana* (fig 3.15), *ardha utkaṭāsana* (fig 3.16) and *pūrṇa utkaṭāsana* (fig 3.17).

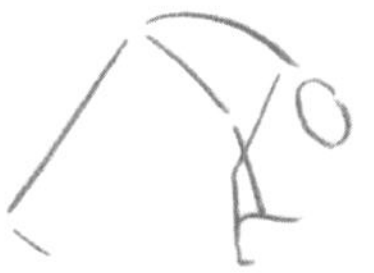

fig 3.14

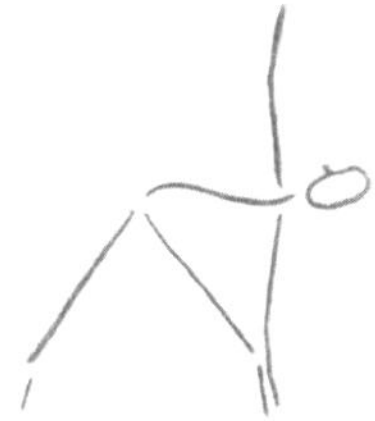

fig 3.15

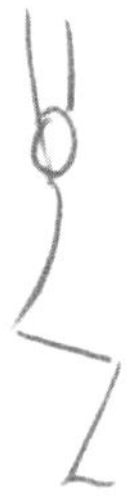

fig 3.16

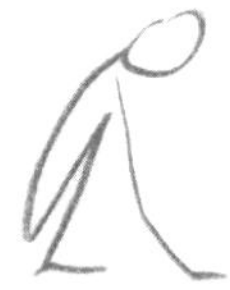

fig 3.17

Kneeling postures

Kneeling postures form a transition between standing and lying and they start from *vajrāsana* (fig 3.18).

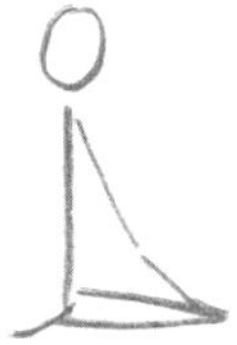

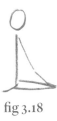

fig 3.18

This posture group is a modern innovation – and here we are primarily referring to kneeling forward bend, cat and perhaps even downward-facing dog[10] (when entered into from a kneeling position). In kneeling postures, we close the eyes and begin to move with more internal awareness. They still offer good freedom of movement so help us to refine the breath and move the body.

Lying postures

Lying postures come next; they allow us to rest after the standing work. They start from *ūrdhva mukha samasthiti* (upward facing *samasthiti,* fig 3.19)

fig 3.19

10. It may seem strange to classify downward-facing dog as a kneeling posture. The reason for this anomaly is that we classify postures from their starting point. Our most common starting point for entering into downward-facing dog is kneeling. If we start the posture from standing, for example from uttānāsana, then we classify it as a standing posture – and this was the traditional classification from Krishnamacharya.

Because the back is fully supported by the ground when lying down, it is harder to damage your back by sudden movements against gravity. With the back stable, lying postures are also excellent for really stretching the legs (often, people try too hard to stretch their legs in standing postures; in a stiff body this has the potential to harm the back). Here we can also begin to work with longer stays in postures and perhaps develop breathing ratios to challenge the breath. Examples include:

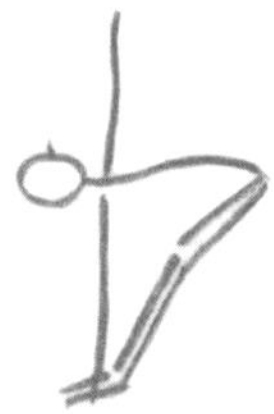

fig 3.20

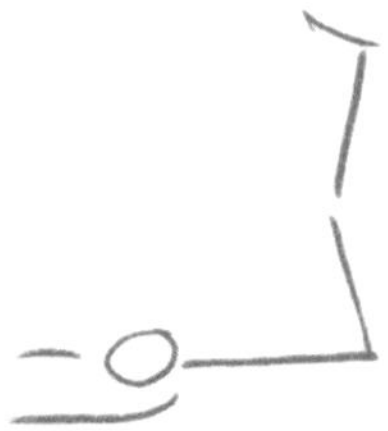

fig 3.21

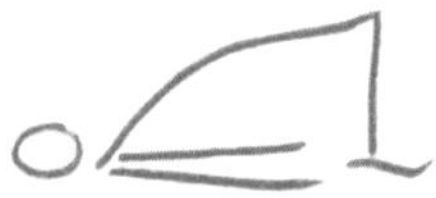

fig 3.22

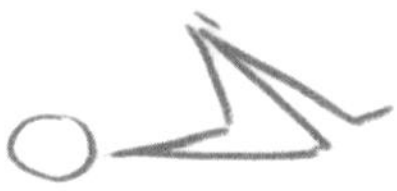

fig 3.23

Inverted postures

Inverted postures are taken deep in the practice, with plenty of preparation – both physical and psychological. Inverting the body is far from our normal upright position and consequently adequate preparation is required. We are primarily talking here about *śīrṣāsana* (headstand, fig 3.24) and *sarvāṅgāsana* (shoulderstand, fig 3.25) – the so-called king and queen of all yoga postures. These postures are taken statically so we can really challenge and cultivate the breath. However, by moving the legs into different positions (e.g. fig 3.26), and even rotating or flexing the spine, headstand and shoulderstand can also include dynamic elements. If you are going to work with both postures, it is usual to perform headstand first. This is because shoulderstand lengthens the neck and thus acts as something of a counterposture here.

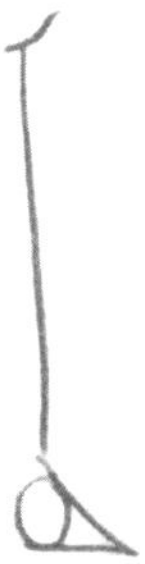

fig 3.24

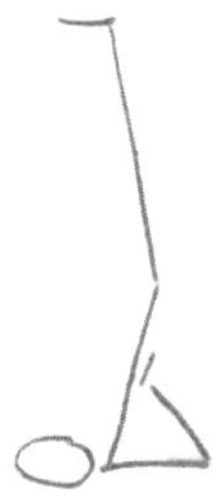

fig 3.25

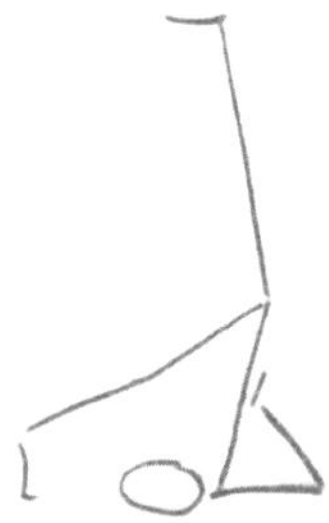

fig 3.26

Backward bends

Here, we focus on prone backward bends such as cobra (*bhujaṅgāsana*) and locust (*śalabhāsana*), which start from *adhomukha samasthiti* (lying on the front, fig 3.27).

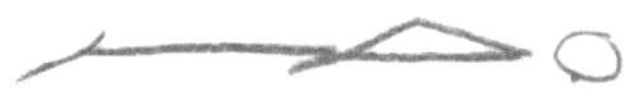

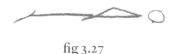

fig 3.27

It is easy for the front of the body to feel compressed after shoulderstand – and even more so after plough (*halāsana*) – so prone backward bends are good counterpostures as they stretch and open the front of the body. Such backward bends do not generally require a huge amount of flexibility; they work more on strengthening the back rather than promoting a lot of movement. They provide an important counterbalance to the strains of modern life where we are often slumped at desks, in driving seats or in badly designed chairs. However, they are also the gateway to backward bends that do require more flexibility – for example, the bow (*dhanurāsana,* fig 3.28) – which are also included in this posture group.

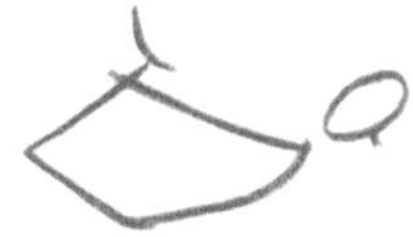

fig 3.28

Seated postures

Because the pelvis is anchored against the floor (or block), seated postures require the most flexibility in the hips, legs and spine; hence as a group they come last. They also encourage deep introspection and are an obvious transition to prāṇāyāma and/or seated meditation. Seated āsana work is at the heart of many yoga practices, and adequate preparation and understanding is required – it is easy to damage knees and backs if these postures are not performed with care, attention and sensitivity. Examples include *jānu śīrṣāsana* (fig 3.29), *ardha matsyendrāsana* (fig 3.30) and *paścimatānāsana* (fig 3.31).

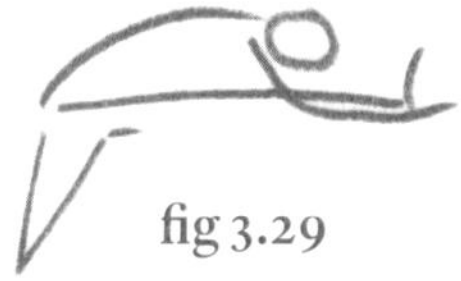

fig 3.29

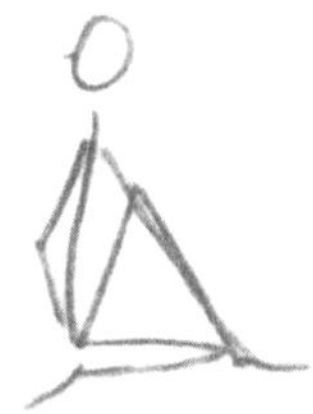

fig 3.30

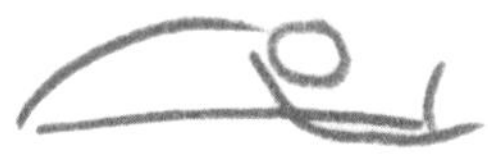

fig 3.31

Although seated postures are the last group, we usually finish with some counterposture – for example, kneeling forward bends or lying on the back and taking some *dvi pāda pītham*. These final counterpostures are not included in the SKLIBS model, but in practice, are almost always present to ensure smooth transition to what follows.

Alternative *vinyāsa krama*

At the beginning of this section, we presented SKLIBS as the default order for an āsana sequence. However, it might well be that we don't want to practise postures from all of the various groups. We may not include inversions in every practice as they require a reasonable amount of time to adequately prepare for. So by dropping inversions, we practice SKLBS. With even less time, we may wish to drop the seated work at the end: SKLB. And perhaps at its most simple, gentle and therapeutic, a practice might simply be KL, like the *pratikriyā* sequence shown on the next page. This sequence, designed by Paul Harvey, is an ideal home practice which can be done in ten minutes and works well for most people. In this practice (see fig 3.32 on next page), each posture is repeated four times.

Take into account the time of day, and your energy levels; if you are practising in the evening after work or when you are very tired, starting lying down can be both restful and energising. Some lying movements can actually build the energy to make standing work more possible. It is also sometimes useful to finish in *samasthiti* – standing with attention and eyes open. This allows us to review the practice and take some transition time before moving on with our day. It is worth reiterating: there are no rules, only principles to guide us. The key things to consider are what precedes the practice and what activities will follow; and to take account of the level of the practitioner, their energy levels, and their general wellbeing. Creating practices is like learning to cook – there is some experimentation, some flexibility, and we can change things for different times, people or occasions. This is the *viniyoga* of sequencing.

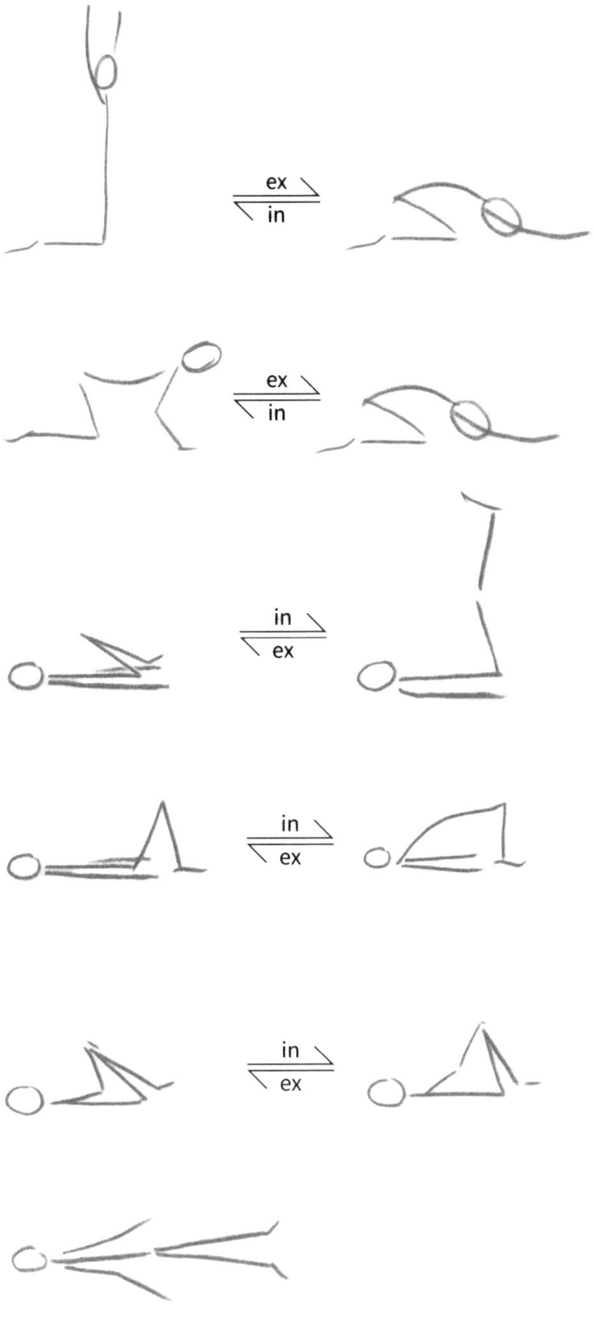

fig 3.32

Chapter 4

हेयं दुःखमनागतम् ।

Yoga and Wellness: A Therapeutic Model

YS 2.16 heyaṃ duḥkham anāgataṃ

Avoid future suffering

Here Patañjali asserts our agency: we do have some element of control and volition, and we are not simply passive victims of fate. While it is impossible to control all future events and experiences, we are at least able to consider how our current actions and thoughts impact on our future. *Heya* means 'that which is to be avoided' while *anāgataṃ* means 'yet to come'. This sūtra is about living in a way that minimises future suffering (*duḥkha*). The *Bhagavad Gītā* defines yoga as 'skill in action' – we practise yoga by most elegantly engaging with our experiences as they arise. By reducing our tendencies to compound our problems, this sort of skilful living helps us to reduce the suffering yet to come.

Unfortunately, many situations are made considerably worse by inappropriate coping mechanisms, unthinking reactions or redundant habits. Like a polluting, un-tuned engine whose carbon emissions are high, unskilful actions leave unwanted residue which continues to reverberate, causing more confusion, delusion and suffering both for ourselves and for others. Can we reduce our 'karmic emissions' to a level whereby we tread lightly on this Earth and leave it – and our relationships – in a better place?

Suffering: *Duḥkha* and its causes

YS 2.15 pariṇāma-tāpa-saṃskāra-duḥkhair guṇa-vṛtti-virodhāc ca duḥkham eva sarvaṃ vivekinaḥ

For those with discrimination, suffering is to be found everywhere due to change (pariṇāma), pain (tāpa) and habits (saṃskāra) and also because the mind is in constant flux due to the guṇa

The starting point for all classical Indian philosophy is *duḥkha,* which is often translated as 'suffering'. But the way our suffering is described and resolved in Indian philosophy is highly nuanced; indeed 'suffering' is too broad a term to do justice to the Sanskrit, and its resolution is not simply anaesthetising ourselves to all pain. The word itself is made up of two syllables: *dus*[1] and *kha*. When used as a prefix, *dus* means 'unfavourable', 'unpleasant' or 'bad'. And the syllable *kha* represents the element of space; here, specifically, the space in our heart, or emotional body. It is said that when energy does not circulate well and we feel 'stuck' we experience *duḥkha* because there is a blockage. Such blockages arise due to past actions, residue that has accumulated and now impedes free flow. One way of resolving this *duḥkha* is to cultivate a feeling of spaciousness (in Sanskrit this is called *sukha*) by removing such blockages whether they are physical, emotional or psychological.

The relationship between the experience of *duḥkha* and our past actions is very important to understand. These actions include our thoughts and emotions as well as our physical actions, because the way we think and feel now is dependent on the way we thought and felt yesterday, and this colours our experience of current events. Actions that we have taken in the past will naturally have consequences, favourable or otherwise, in the present and future. But equally the psychology behind those actions, the motives and thought processes, will impact on how we relate to

1. In Sanskrit, the 's' changes to an 'ḥ' when followed by the 'k' in *duḥkha*.

our lives as they unfold. Are we bitter, resigned, carefree, indifferent, happy or lazy? The residue of thoughts and actions (*karma-āśaya*) are the seeds for future experiences. This is why *karma* (which means both an action and also that action's consequences) is such a central theme of classical Indian philosophy; we cannot understand *duḥkha* without some appreciation of *karma*.

The philosophy of Sāṃkhya, sometimes seen as the sister to Patañjali's Yoga Sūtra, was codified roughly 1,600 years ago by Īśvara Kṛṣṇa in his classic work, *Sāṃkhya Kārikā* ('Verses on Sāṃkhya'). The text starts by stating that the purpose of Sāṃkhya is the resolution of three types of *duḥkha*. The three types are understood to be:

- *ādhyātmika* – suffering caused by oneself
- *ādhibhautika* – suffering caused by other creatures
- *ādhidaivika* – suffering caused by divine forces

His solution to the problem of *duḥkha* is discriminative knowledge (which is called *viveka* in the Yoga Sūtra): the cultivation of insight that cuts through illusions and sets us free. Only this discriminative knowledge is a certain cure for *duḥkha* he says; all other remedies are subject to uncertainty or decay.[2] Careful investigation into both the nature of ourselves and the nature of all that surrounds us is the way out of the maze of *duḥkha*. Thus for Īśvara Kṛṣṇa, the only surefire resolution is philosophical enquiry and the gradual reshaping of our habitual understanding of the world. This necessitates a new way of thinking and being.

In YS 2.15, Patañjali also divides *duḥkha* into three types, but they are presented in a slightly different way than in the *Sāṃkhya Kārikā*. Patañjali says that *duḥkha* is inevitable because of the fluctuating nature of the *guṇa*.[3] As we have seen, the *guṇa* are the essence of not just the entire phenomenal world, but most importantly, the very nature of our minds. When our actions are strongly coloured by excess *rajas* or *tamas*, and are thereby characterised by inappropriate desire and agitation (*rajas*) or by dullness,

2. 'Uncertainty' implies that our subjective conclusions are not foolproof, and 'decay' suggests the teaching of tradition is subject to change over time: it easily degenerates and is corrupted. Here, rigorous philosophical reasoning is the preferred method.

3. See Chapter 7 for further discussion on the *guṇa*.

delusion and rigidity (*tamas*), then their consequences will have some of these qualities too.

The first type of *duḥkha* Patañjali refers to is called *pariṇāma duḥkha*. The dance of the *guṇa* ensures that nothing is permanent; change (*pariṇāma*) means we suffer from *pariṇāma duḥkha* – the emotional constriction that arises when what we would like to remain, changes. A beautiful ripe fruit will decay and become rotten; an enjoyable meal of excess can result in tummy problems or a headache the next day. Everything moves, sometimes slowly and sometimes very quickly, and even moments of great beauty and happiness are tinged with the poignancy of knowing that they will end. And of course, our minds also change – sometimes we are clear and at others, consumed by anxiety, worry or remorse and regret.

Whilst *pariṇāma duḥkha* is the result of change, its flipside, *saṃskāra duḥkha*, is the result of our tendency to create and maintain habitual ways of thinking, feeling and acting. Our minds love to create habits, to move down well-worn tracks of thinking and being. These patterns of habit are called *saṃskāra*, and our *saṃskāra* will naturally create certain consequences, as thoughts solidify into actions and actions solidify into our ways of living. The repetition of small *saṃskāra* can have big consequences as their effects accumulate.

Of course not all *saṃskāra* are small. We can say that any type of suffering which results from our patterning and our habits, however large or trivial, is *saṃskāra duḥkha*. It is also worth remembering that *saṃskāra duḥkha* can arise out of simply being stuck in a habit that is no longer appropriate. Where once a strategy worked, now it has become redundant and is causing unhappiness – either to us or to others.

The third type of *duḥkha* to which Patañjali refers is *tāpa duḥkha*. *Tāpa* comes from the root *tap*, meaning 'to heat'. It is the suffering which arises from pain, from the myriad forms of discomfort, be they physical (standing on a nail, being bitten by an animal, being too hot or too cold) or emotional/psychological (being thwarted, unfulfilled, rejected, bored, angry). Thus *tāpa duḥkha* comes from the pain arising from our senses and their connection to our minds, particularly related to our desires and expectations. We can subdivide *tāpa duḥkha* into the three types that are spoken about in the *Sāṃkhya Kārikā*: *ādhyātmika* (caused by myself), *ādhibhautika* (caused by other creatures), and *ādhidaivika* (caused by divine forces).[4] Patañjali elaborates the model of *duḥkha* to include suffering arising from natural change and suffering arising from habitual patterns:

Patañjali:	***pariṇāma duḥkha***	***tāpa duḥkha***	***saṃskāra duḥkha***
	Suffering caused by change	Suffering caused by pain ↓	Suffering caused by habit
Īśvara Kṛṣṇa:		***ādhyātmika*** – caused by oneself ***ādhibhautika*** – caused by other creatures ***ādhidaivika*** – caused by divine forces	

What suffering can we avoid?

Can we avoid all *duḥkha*? It is impossible (and undesirable) to feel no pain as long as we are alive. Pain acts as a warning and is therefore often very useful. However, the *duḥkha* we are considering is neither helpful nor desirable: it is the consequence of misunderstanding and unskilful action. Some *duḥkha* is conscious – we *know* that we are suffering – but at other times, it is unconscious. Often, we are unaware of what we are carrying, of how we think, and how this may colour our perceptions. Many people anaesthetise themselves with food, alcohol, drugs, sex or the internet as a way of remaining unconscious to their own suffering. Someone in a coma may well not experience the suffering of a conscious person, but Patañjali does not advocate shutting down to resolve pain. Instead he acknowledges

4. This observation has come from Edwin Bryant, *The Yoga Sūtra of Patanjali* (North Point Press, 2013), p. 207 who references Vyāsa here.

there are certain types of *duḥkha* that we can avoid and that it's very possible to not contribute to future frustrations and suffering by how we think and act right now. In essence: when you are in a hole, stop digging.

Of course, there may be *duḥkha* coming to us which we can do nothing about; it would be naive to suggest that we can still retain feelings like pleasure and joy and yet totally eradicate all experience of pain. The loss of a loved one will naturally affect us; however, the host of thoughts that may go alongside any such event ("I wish it were otherwise", "I should have done this or that", "What is to become of me?" and so on) will be significantly reduced as we refine our relationship to and experience of *duḥkha*. How we experience that pain, how we understand it, and how we most elegantly deal with it, are the subjects at the heart of the yoga project. And in this quest, we must first ask: what is it that keeps producing *duḥkha*? What creates and maintains our suffering? We must turn our attention to *hetu,* the cause.

Creating and maintaining our suffering

YS 2.17 draṣṭṛ-dṛśyayoḥ saṃyoga heya-hetuḥ

Confusing the source of perception with the objects of perception is the root of suffering

In any experience, there is always the event itself and then our understanding of and reaction to the event. Some events are difficult, some are pleasant; however, the inability to distinguish an event from our reactions to it is the source of much unnecessary anguish.

Avidyā[5] is this state of confusion. The term comprises '*vidyā*', meaning 'to know' (and is related to English words like 'vision' and 'video'), and the prefix '*a*', which implies the opposite. However, although *avidyā* literally means 'not knowing' or 'not seeing', it is more than simply wilful blindness. We can be aware that we can't see something but when we are in a state of *avidyā,* we cannot see *because we see something else*. Our misunderstanding of a situation

5. For a more detailed discussion of *avidyā* and *saṃyoga* see Chapter 8.

obscures a deeper reality. *Avidyā* is, therefore, by its very nature, unconscious: if we know we can't see something we are not in a state of *avidyā*, but one of conscious ignorance.

In YS 2.17, Patañjali goes even deeper into the notion of *avidyā*. He uses the term *saṃyoga* almost synonymously with *avidyā*, saying that it is this *saṃyoga* that is the cause (*hetu*) of our suffering. Whereas *avidyā* is more abstract and theoretical, *saṃyoga* is its embodied state; it is how we actually experience *avidyā*. *Saṃyoga* is 'complete joining', the bodily experience of mixed-up confusion, where we cannot make subtle distinctions because different elements are so enmeshed with each other that they look like a single event. In YS 2.17, Patañjali proposes that the inability to distinguish our thoughts and perceptions (*dṛśya*[6]) from a pure awareness utterly devoid of characteristics (*draṣṭṛ*[7]) is at the very heart of the human predicament; this is the experience of *avidyā* at its most profound. By utterly identifying with the ephemeral contents of our consciousness, we mistake ourselves for the movie that we are in: the actor completely identifies with the role. As we have discussed in Chapter 2, this is our normal state and it dooms us to the endless cycle of mistakes and confusion that cause and maintain *duḥkha*.

Although *saṃyoga* and *avidyā* are defined by Patañjali in profound philosophical terms, we find *saṃyoga* and *avidyā* present in many everyday situations – for example, a beginner to yoga will often be unable to distinguish subtle movements in their own body and feel the whole body moving like a single block. In relationships too, we may confuse our thoughts and projections for another's – who we think we are is blurred with our fantasies about another person. Once we start noticing, we find *saṃyoga* everywhere and its resolution (clarifying and making appropriate distinctions) can bring about a feeling of freedom and space in many difficult situations. Once again, the most profound philosophical understandings of the Yoga Sūtra are also reflected in our everyday lived experience.

6. A synonym for *citta*.

7. A synonym for *cit* or *puruṣa*.

Hāna: The space of liberation

YS 2.25 tad-abhāvāt saṃyoga-abhāvo hānaṃ tad-dṛśeḥ kaivalyaṃ

As this tendency diminishes, the path to freedom develops

The Roman philosopher Seneca famously said: "If one does not know to which port one is sailing, no wind is favourable." Having already analysed how and why we suffer, and also what maintains this suffering, in YS 2.25 Patañjali presents his solution. As we have seen in Chapter 1, it is a popular notion that the goal of all yoga is union with the Divine, or a merging with a greater reality. Though this may be the case in some traditions, Patañjali's goal is rather different. His goal – indeed, he claims, the goal of all experience – is to disentangle oneself from the enmeshment and identification with the contents of our minds. He describes this in YS 2.25 as *abhāva* (removal) of *saṃyoga* (enmeshment). Only through this practice of disentangling can one achieve true freedom or *kaivalya*.

Kaivalya literally translates as 'alone-ness', which on the surface may sound undesirable. However, what Patañjali means here is something positive: a freedom that arises from clarification between the essence of our Being and the projections of our minds. Instead of a merging, there is a differentiation; and although it may seem counterintuitive, it is this very differentiation which brings wholeness and a spaciousness. This is the 'path to freedom', the escape route (*hāna*). Enmeshment, *saṃyoga*, is the opposite condition – where we are compromised and restricted, adding to our own suffering unconsciously.

Upāya: The means

YS 2.26 viveka-khyātir aviplavā hānopāyaḥ

Consistent discernment is the means to overcoming (saṃyoga/avidyā)

There are many arenas in which we become entangled; each of our many facets and layers has the potential to become mired in *avidyā*. As *saṃyoga* diminishes, the escape route (*hānaṃ*) becomes clearer – through cultivation of *viveka khyātir*, discriminative awareness. In his famous *aṣṭāṅga yoga*, Patañjali describes eight arenas, and therefore eight types of practice, for the cultivation of this discriminative awareness. These practices are called *upāya* – the means. By addressing these many layers, from the interpersonal through to the subtlest aspects of mind, Patañjali ensures that the yoga project is systemic and multi-dimensional.

The eight limbs of yoga each address a different sort of *saṃyoga* by cultivating spaciousness and clarity (*sattva*), at that level. Although some practices help to prepare for others by providing a stable support, they are not to be thought of as purely sequential but rather as developing simultaneously. The eight limbs of yoga provide support and give direction to each other so that the whole of our Being is increasingly experienced as light, free and spacious. Five of the eight limbs can be thought of as more external; these are discussed at the end of Chapter 2 of the Yoga Sūtra. The three which are seen as more internal are discussed at the beginning of Chapter 3 of the Yoga Sūtra.

External limbs: *bahir-aṅgaṃ*

- *Yama* is concerned with freedom in relationship. We explore these further in Chapter 11.
- *Niyama* is concerned with freedom from our destructive and unhelpful habits. We explore these further in Chapters 12 and 13.
- *Āsana* brings freedom to the body, encouraging lightness, stability and health. We explore this further in Chapter 9.

- *Prāṇāyāma* refines our patterns of breathing and brings an extraordinary sensitivity to the flow of the breath and therefore our vital energy (*prāṇa*). We explore this further in Chapter 10.
- *Pratyāhāra* frees us from the tyranny of our senses and gives us choice about how we engage with sensuality. We explore this further in Chapter 14.

Internal limbs: *antar-aṅgaṃ*

- *Dhāraṇā* focuses our attention on a single object, thereby cultivating mental stability and freedom from distraction.
- *Dhyānam* deepens that focus and enables true insight and freedom from mental projections.
- *Samādhi* frees us from habitual self-centredness, allowing new and profound insights to arise. We explore all of these three practices in Chapter 13.

These last three limbs are collectively known as *saṃyama*, the process of deepening a meditative practice. In their purest form, they are aimed at clarifying the distinction between the subtlest aspects of our consciousness and the pure empty awareness of *puruṣa*, and are therefore seen as advanced practices which require considerable stability and preparation. However, it is important not to dismiss *saṃyama* as too esoteric and therefore irrelevant. We explore some practical means of applying the principles of *saṃyama* in a simple and accessible way in Chapter 15.

Sādhana: Preparation and counterposture

In Chapter 3 we considered how the careful construction of a practice is fundamental to this approach. Any activity that requires a number of steps – cooking, painting or building – requires *vinyāsa krama,* the intelligent ordering of those steps. Two essential aspects of *vinyāsa krama* in āsana and prāṇāyāma are preparation and counterposture. In Sanskrit, *pūrvāṅga* means 'prior, preparatory parts'; it is the way we skilfully move towards a goal – it is the preparation. The word *pratikriyāsana* tells us something of the qualities of counterposture. *Prati* means 'against', or 'opposite'; *kriyā* means 'action' and so *pratikriyāsana* literally means 'opposite action; posture'. Both *pūrvāṅga* and *pratikriyā* will help us 'anticipate and avoid future suffering'.

Pūrvāṅga: Preparation

As any painter and decorator will tell you, the quality of the preparation will define the quality of the end product. If you skimp on the preparation, even though a job may look good initially, it will deteriorate and show itself as second-rate soon enough. Similarly, the quality of the preparation in āsana and prāṇāyāma, in both the short and the long term, will define the quality and experience of a posture or technique. Without adequate preparation, a posture might not be well executed or integrated into the practice, and there will also be considerably greater chances of injury.

In some classes, students are taught to warm up prior to the yoga class. Desikachar always stated that the preparation should be part of the actual practice – there is no need for 'pre-yoga warm-ups'. A useful principle is that we move from symmetrical, simple and dynamic postures to postures which are more complex. We slowly build up the intensity so that the body, breath and attention are all brought into an alignment and can thereby work together with maximum integrity.

For example, before we work with a static asymmetrical standing posture, we would prepare with some dynamic, symmetrical work which warms and mobilises the body, engages our attention and prepares the breath for deep and slow breathing (fig 4.1).

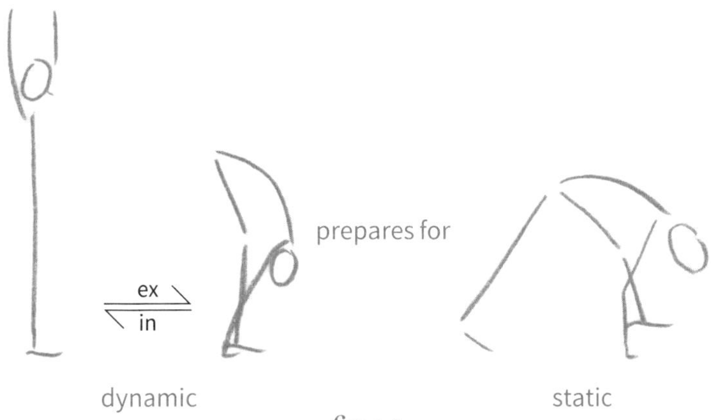

fig 4.1

As we have already seen in Chapter 3, the art of *vinyāsa krama* uses groups of postures to help prepare us for other groups. So standing postures will help to prepare us for more complex postures deeper in the practice; lying postures can help for seated postures (because they can safely stretch the backs of the legs). And in general, work with the body (āsana) will prepare us for static work with the breath (prāṇāyāma) which in turn prepares us for still seated meditation practices (*dhyāna*).

When our goal is a complex backbend, we should prepare with some gentler backbends; similarly, complex twists require simple twists as preparation. Generally speaking, standing backward bends (for example, the warrior, *vīrabhadrāsana* 1, fig 4.2), prepare us for more challenging prone backward bends (for example, the bow, *dhanurāsana*, fig 4.3).

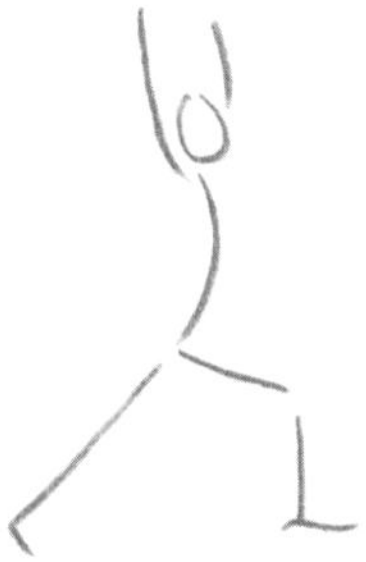

prepares for

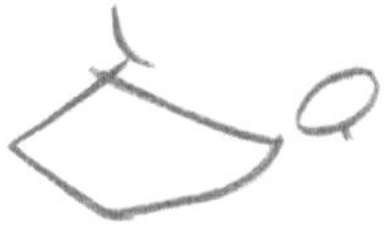

fig 4.2

fig 4.3

Similarly, standing forward bends (standing forward bend, *uttānāsana*; flank forward bend, *pārśva uttānāsana,* fig 4.4; and even the full squat, *utkaṭāsana*) can prepare for seated forward bends (*jānu śīrṣāsana,* fig 4.5 or *paścimatānāsana*) later in the practice.

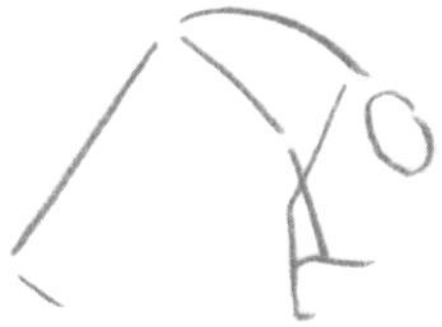

prepares for

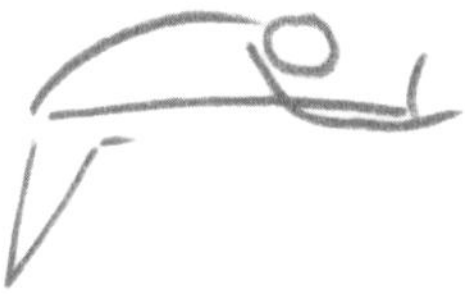

fig 4.4

fig 4.5

A seated twist (usually static, fig 4.7) will be helped by a standing twist (fig 4.6, often dynamic) and a lying twist (perhaps dynamic and static). Of course, not everyone will need the same amount of preparation: the body temperature, time of the day and many other variables will mean that sometimes more and sometimes less preparation is required.

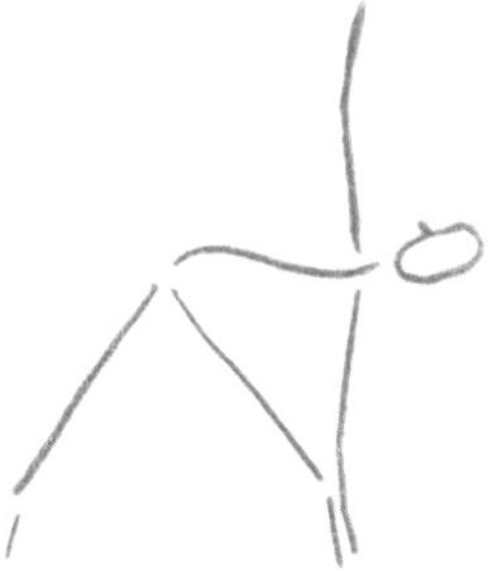

prepares for

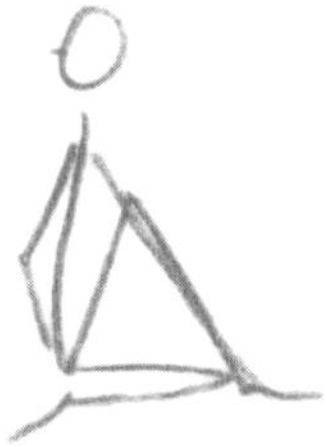

fig 4.6

fig 4.7

Pratikriyāsana: Counterposture

Desikachar was fond of telling a story – perhaps apocryphal – about when he was a young boy and was encouraged by his brothers to climb a palm tree for coconuts. He got up fine, but once up wasn't sure how to get down! This principle of understanding the route down, a sort of 'opposite action', is the basis of counterposture. In fact, Desikachar emphasised the importance of being able to perform a counterposture before attempting the main posture. An example of this is the shoulderstand (fig 4.8). Desikachar insisted that if you are unable to comfortably perform the counterposture – in this case dynamic cobra while sweeping the arms (fig 4.9) – then you should not attempt the posture. The counterposture thereby becomes a useful check: if you cannot do it properly, then do not attempt the posture.

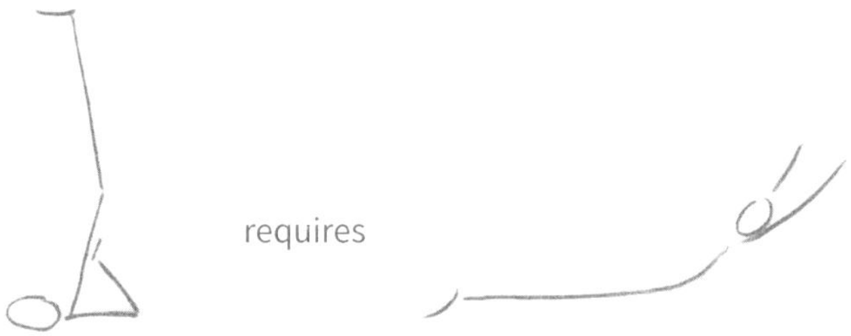

fig 4.8 fig 4.9

As we have seen, the theory of *karma* says that every action we take, including thoughts, has consequences. Some of these consequences may be positive, some less so. When we perform an āsana, the body and breath are challenged in particular ways and this affects the whole system. Not all of the effects will necessarily be positive; however, with adequate and sensitive counterposture, the negative effects of the posture can be minimised without 'neutralising' all of the positive effects. For example, after performing a number of seated forward bends, although the back has been lengthened and the back of the legs stretched, the hips have been closed for a long time and the lumbar lordosis flattened and reversed. Although we want to keep the feeling of having stretched the back of the body, we might also like to open and move the hips and also slightly arch the back to feel some sense of realignment. So counterpostures might include two-foot support, or kneeling forward bend.

Although there are some general principles, not everyone will need the same counterpostures. One person may need to address a hip stiffness, for someone else their neck may be the issue, or a problem in a shoulder or tightness in the back. As with so much in yoga, what is appropriate depends on the individual – and this, too, may change from day to day.

Not every posture requires a counterposture; we do not want to be continuously bending one way and then the other. Sometimes, we can perform a series of postures together – for example, a series of prone backward bends. It could be that only after the entire series do we need to take some counterposture. Another important principle here is that generally the counterposture is less intense than the main posture, it is not simply a movement in the opposite direction, but rather a gentler (usually dynamic) movement to address specific areas. Where there was compression, a counterposture can gently stretch; where there was holding, a counterposture can move; where there was asymmetry, a counterposture can realign.

Because the counterposture is less intense than the main posture, we also tend to perform it for fewer breaths. A good rule of thumb is that a counterposture should last somewhere between one third and one half of the length of the main posture(s). So, for example, 12 breaths in a lying twist (6 breaths to each side), would entail 4–6 breaths in counterposture. If we worked with a series of forward bends for 30 breaths, we would need 10–15 breaths in counterpostures – and there may be more than one counter posture here (to address different parts of the body).

The importance of forward bends as counterposture

Of all the possible movements of the spine, forward bends are the most useful when it comes to counterposture. Gary Kraftsow[8] likens the forward bend to neutral when we change gears in a car – we have to travel through neutral to move from one gear to another. In the same way, when we move from twists to backward bends, or backward bends to flank stretches, symmetrical forward bends are required. The original shape of the spine in an embryo is flexion, so you could say that forward bends return the spine to its 'default setting' – they 'return us to ourselves'.

Forward bends require an exhalation, and exhalation is linked to letting go of the past. Often when we have just succeeded in doing something very difficult, or we want to move on from a situation, we breathe a sigh of relief; an exhalation helps us to move forward. Exhales have a psychologically soothing effect and help us 'wipe the blackboard clean'. They clear what has accumulated and make a space to receive something new. Thus, both in terms of form and breath, forward bends are very useful as counterpostures.

We use a convenient acronym to remember the attributes of good counterposture – DOES:

- **D**ynamic: counterpostures are best performed dynamically. Movements free up areas of stiffness and holding, and also ease the breath. Dynamic work generally requires less effort than holding a posture statically, as tension does not build up in the same way.
- **O**pposite: counterpostures open where the body has been closed and close where the body has been open.
- **E**asy: the counterposture should be less demanding than the main posture. Counterpostures do not bounce you from one extreme to another; they gently work in an opposing direction to bring realignment and balance.
- **S**ymmetrical: generally speaking, symmetrical postures

8. Gary Kraftsow, *Yoga for Transformation: Ancient Teachings and Practices for Healing the Body, Mind, and Heart* (Arkana, 2002), p. 67.

are psychologically containing. They are simple, less complicated and return the body to balance.

Of course there may be exceptions to this, but these are useful guiding principles for us to consider when thinking about *pratikriyāsana*.

Chapter 5

अभ्यासवैराग्याभ्यां तन्निरोधः ।

The Essential Method

YS 1.12 abhyāsa vairāgyābhyāṃ tan nirodhaḥ

Containing the mind requires the cultivation of both stability and openness

We have already looked at the concept of *nirodha* in Chapter 2 and discussed how it is part of both the process and the goal of yoga. In YS 1.12 Patañjali provides a concrete statement of how to reach the state of *nirodha*, offering us an essential methodology in the form of *abhyāsa* and *vairāgya*. *Abhyāsa* suggests practice and discipline. It means 'to travel forwards towards a goal' and, in this case, indicates the necessity for stability and continuity of practice in pursuit of the state of yoga. However, *abhyāsa* needs a partner lest it becomes over-zealous and rigid; this partner is *vairāgya*.

Although often translated as 'detachment' (which seems rather aloof and indifferent), *vairāgya* is a kind of radical 'non-stick openness'. Its literal meaning is 'moving away from (*vi-*) desire (*rāga*)'. But only viewing it as 'turning away' can trap us in an unhealthy polarity, constantly oscillating between on/off, yes/no, will I/won't I. This all too often ends in disappointment and failure. Instead, *vairāgya* can be thought of as cultivating an open space in which new possibilities can arise. We move away from the push/pull duality and towards a place where we have the freedom to use the supports of *abhyāsa* to disengage from that which blocks us. *Vairāgya* can be seen as 'turning towards' rather than 'turning away' from something: from defensiveness to openness, from rejecting to embracing. This understanding of *vairāgya* allows us to be really touched by life, to experience it fully without clutching at it, holding on, or becoming addicted, defensive or reactive. These two fundamental elements, *abhyāsa* and *vairāgya*, lie at the heart of the yoga method; we could even say that they *are* the yoga method and everything else is elaboration. Just as a bird needs two wings to fly, *abhyāsa* and *vairāgya* complement each other and both are essential in helping us to move towards a state of yoga.

Defining *abhyāsa*

YS 1.13 tatra sthitau yatno'bhyāsaḥ

Abhyāsa is the effort to be stable there (in a state of nirodha)

In YS 1.13, Patañjali defines what he means by *abhyāsa*: "the effort (*yatna*) to be stable (*sthiti*) there (in a state of *nirodha*)". There are two key concepts here: effort and stability. The effort itself needs to be stable, and also to produce stability. Of course, practice requires effort, but Herculean effort performed intermittently is not *abhyāsa*. *Abhyāsa* necessitates consistent, committed and steadfast practice; the most important word in this sūtra is *sthiti* – stability. Furthermore, stability is both the support and the direction: the measure of this effort (*abhyāsa*) is the stability it brings. Stability therefore is both in the quality of the effort and is also its fruit.

We could say that *abhyāsa* is 'the effort to put our supports in place'. The supports will help us fly. This effort is not to be done half-heartedly; it requires a steady application of will, and a persistence that is neither rigid and dogmatic on the one hand, nor lacking in vigour and purpose on the other. It is relatively easy to reach a state of clarity – but it will be ephemeral and unstable if it is not well grounded. *Abhyāsa* is about not slipping and this often requires us to swim upstream a little, to challenge ourselves – always from a place of stability. Too often, yoga is associated with a kind of New Age airiness that can create great experiences that do not last. *Abhyāsa* is about cultivating traits, and not simply states. Although it is sometimes not a popular message, stability and discipline lie at the very heart of the yoga tradition.

YS 1.14 sa tu dīrgha-kāla-nairantarya-satkāra-ādarā-āsevito dṛḍha-bhūmiḥ

Abhyāsa takes a long time, needs to be consistent, and performed with integrity and enthusiasm before it is firmly established

Here, Patañjali develops his definition of *abhyāsa* by describing the qualities of this effort. In order to cultivate (*āsevito*) stability (*dṛḍhabhūmiḥ*) we must practise for a long time (*dīrgha-kāla*), without interruption (*nairantarya*), with care and sensitivity (*satkāra*), and with enthusiasm and respect (*ādara*).[1] Let us explore each of these in turn.

Dīrgha-kāla means 'a long time', and *nairantarya* means 'without interruption'. Yoga practice requires 'flying hours' – starting yoga twenty years ago, but only practising occasionally, is not *abhyāsa*! Yoga is a gradual path that requires many years to mature and grow. We can liken it to wearing out the sole of a shoe – you have to travel many miles and the process is gradual, but, as the old saying goes, a journey of a thousand miles begins with a single step. However, this does not mean that the practice has to remain the same throughout the journey. In fact, repeating the same practice can be both limiting and harmful to the body, particularly as we age over the years.

Although much is made in āsana teaching about safety, if one listens to the responses of the body, starts simply and then gradually adds intensity and depth in careful steps then the matter is largely common sense. This long-term approach to yoga practice therefore needs to be cultivated with care and sensitivity, listening to the body and its responses. We need authenticity (*satkāra*) in our practice and awareness of our own responses. There also needs to be some zeal and challenge (*ādara*) – we must sometimes approach our edge (physical, mental, emotional), otherwise the practice never deepens and matures. At its most dubious, modern yoga practice can tend to swing between two extremes – either a slavish adherence to a fixed form or

1. The word *ādara* appears in editions of the Yoga Sūtra which have originated from the teachings of Krishnamacharya, but not in other editions of the text. Also in his commentary, Vyāsa refers to the other qualities, *dīrghakāla, nairantarya, satkāra*, but not to *ādara*. This leads us to hypothesise that it was added by Krishnamacharya.

a rather random approach where is there is little structure or intelligent methodology (and so progress is rather haphazard).

Another meaning of the term yoga is 'to reach a point we have not reached before',[2] and in this context, the practice should develop in steps. This is known as *yoga-kṣema*. Yoga here refers to the introduction of new elements into the practice. *Kṣema* refers to the *sthiti* elements – that is to say, the maintenance of the practice and integration of these new steps, with sensitivity towards the body's responses. If something can be integrated without any problems for some time, then there is the possibility of taking another step. If not, the practice needs to be revised. Clearly this implies regular practice.

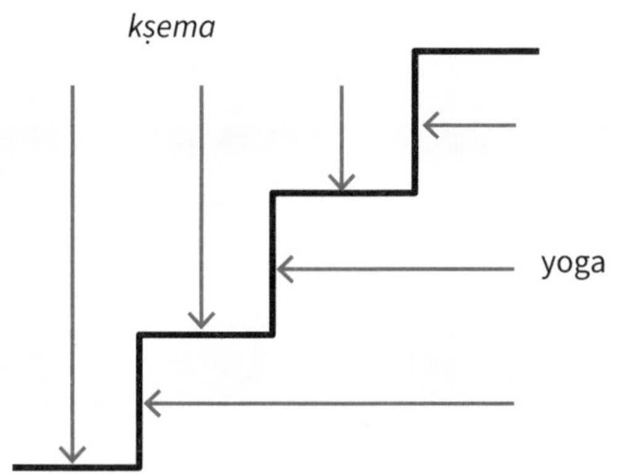

This is where the occasional group class can be problematic. If practices are introduced without checking and integrating the preliminary steps, difficulties may arise. For example, sometimes students are taught to retain their breath in prāṇāyāma before they have developed sufficient ability to simply inhale and exhale. Without creating the foundations by establishing a long and subtle breath, retention of the breath may be experienced as stressful and unsustainable.

Which is more difficult: yoga or *kṣema*? Do we become attached to the familiarity and security of our regular

2. TKV Desikachar, *Religiousness in Yoga* p 2.

practice and find it hard to introduce new elements, or do we like new aspects of practice, but find it hard to maintain the form of a practice consistently? For most of us, it is relatively easy to start something new; the challenge is to maintain the practice regularly and consistently.

This leads us to the issue of regular practice *without interruption*, of maintaining continuity (*nairantarya*). Yoga was traditionally a daily practice and the regular practice provided a mirror for our state of being from day to day. Daily practice is certainly ideal, but we have to be realistic and may have to revise our expectations. However, it is important to maintain some sense of continuity: yoga is a training and the body and the mind need time and regularity to respond. Although attending a weekly class can be of

'For most of us, it is relatively easy to start something new; the challenge is to maintain the practice regularly and consistently.'

considerable benefit, ultimately the practice needs to be much more regular to have optimum impact on the body and mind. It is far better to practise for a shorter time each day than for one two-hour session once a week, just as it is better to clean your teeth for five minutes each day rather than for an hour on a Sunday!

The need for enthusiasm and respect (*ādara*) points to important attitudes that help to keep the practice potent. Approaching our practice as a chore significantly limits our involvement, so it is important to find a way to look forward to practice. Reflect on the good fortune that we have to live in a place and time where we have the freedom and space to engage with the practice: this is a luxury that many people in the world do not have. Another idea is to dedicate the energy of the practice towards something greater than ourselves, or towards the welfare of others. This embraces the idea of having respect for the practice: it is something special that can touch us deeply if we let it, so we respect it as something precious. When someone first discovers yoga, they may not have the sensitivity or insight to recognise the potential of what they are doing, but as their practice develops it can be like a love affair where the practice offers untold promise, magic and mystery. It is easy to maintain the enthusiasm and respect here – it is as if one becomes enchanted and the practice enlivens all aspects of our lives. But this magic invariably wears off a little at times and we can become stale or uninspired. This is when there is the real challenge of *abhyāsa*: how to maintain the qualities once the honeymoon period is over.

Defining *vairāgya*

YS 1.15 dṛṣṭa-ānuśravika-viṣaya-vitṛṣṇasya vaśīkāra-saṃjñā vairāgyam

Vairāgya requires equanimity to both secular and spiritual pursuits

Although *abhyāsa* is at the heart of the yoga method, on its own it is fundamentally limited. *Abhyāsa* needs *vairāgya*, lest it leads to unbending zeal and becomes a prison. We have seen how *vairāgya* is frequently translated as 'detachment' or 'lack of desire', and indeed, the literal meaning is 'away from desire'. Although *viṣaya-vitṛṣṇasya* means 'an absence of thirst (*vitṛṣṇasya*) towards objects (*viṣaya*)', the really important word in the sūtra is *vaśīkāra* – 'mastery'. This term implies an ability to remain centred, without being knocked off balance and impelled to behave in ways we might later regret. *Vairāgya* is the ability to reside in a space without the compulsion to act; it gives us the freedom to choose how to respond.

Interestingly, Patañjali defines *vairāgya* as applying to both material things *and* spiritual aspirations. The term *dṛṣṭa-ānuśravika* literally means 'the seen (*dṛṣṭa*) and the heard (*ānuśravika*)'. The first term, *dṛṣṭa,* is generally understood to refer to worldly, material objects – things that are tangible and can be seen. The second term, *ānuśravika,* implies less obvious desires, but includes treasures we may hear about from sacred texts – in other words, spiritual treasures, the promise of heaven. It is common to simply impose desires and aspirations from worldly life onto the spiritual domain; we become enamoured not with our car or house but with our abilities in practice or the promise of yogic powers (even if that's just mastering a posture). Nothing really changes; our vanities simply become subtler. Instead, something about our attitude towards our practice, and indeed towards life generally, needs to change. *Vairāgya* invites us to cultivate less expectation about the results.

Simply understanding *vairāgya* as 'detachment' could lead us to become cold, unfeeling and somewhat cut off from life. Instead we could consider *vairāgya* as a state of play that eventually enables a certain mastery (*vaśīkāra*). When we are confident in our ability to 'let be', to not get caught up in desire or aversion, we have achieved a certain level of *vairāgya*. This is neither easy nor instant. First we may need to deliberately turn away from and shun certain experiences in order to protect ourselves from habitual desires, aversions or ways of being. However, as we cultivate a new orientation, we can begin to be more open to experiences without feeling overwhelmed or destabilised. We can therefore see the cultivation of *vairāgya* as a *vinyāsa*: mastery arises only after careful steps which ensure the protection and stability of our fledgling *vairāgya*.[3] Ultimately, the test of *vairāgya* is the ability to let ourselves be touched by life and yet still remain open and innocent.

3. It is generally understood that there are four steps in this process, of which *vaśīkāra* is the last. The first requires deliberate effort to renounce aspects of our lives that generate excessive attachment. The second is a degree of mastery in which one recognises triggers that may entrap us. The third is when mastery has been achieved, but there is still a potential in the mind to be drawn off course. Only in *vaśīkāra* is there profound stability.

YS 1.16 tat paraṃ puruṣa-khyāter guṇa-vaitṛṣṇyam

The highest vairāgya arises when we remain unreactive to all of prakṛti, and we intuit the pure awareness of puruṣa

Which is most important: *abhyāsa* or *vairāgya*? As is often the case, their order in the Yoga Sūtra is significant: *abhyāsa* comes before *vairāgya*. We have to start with some *abhyāsa*. But the Yoga Sūtra suggests that ultimately it is the cultivation of *vairāgya* that will take us to the highest stages of yoga. In fact, Patañjali states that the highest *vairāgya,* where we have no thirst for the *guṇa* themselves (*guṇa-vaitṛṣṇyam*), will only come from a profound vision of our deepest nature (*puruṣa-khyāti*). This is not surprising: the more we have confidence in our own profound nature, something that transcends mundane experience, the more we can be open and responsive to the world around us without the need for defensiveness and fear. This seems to be a radical path of freedom: not freedom *from* the world, but freedom *within* the world.

Sādhana: *Abhyāsa* and *vairāgya* in āsana and prāṇāyāma

Let us take some practical examples to see how we can apply the idea of 'putting support in place' – our interpretation of Patañjali's definition of *abhyāsa*. In any āsana, we could ask: what do we need to do, to ensure that the posture is stable and supported? There needs to be some effort and commitment, skilfully applied, and the ability to know when, and how, to release the body. Yoga postures and their myriad variations can often deliberately put the body into unusual configurations where stability is compromised and challenged.

In this variation of *dvi pāda pīṭham* (fig 5.1), we start in *supta baddha konāsana*, with the soles of the feet together and the hips open.

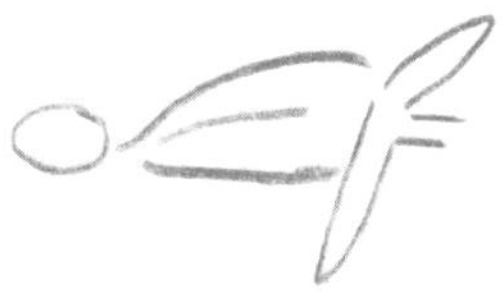

fig 5.1

When we enter the posture, by raising the hips off the floor, the pelvis can feel quite unstable as it is not obviously 'held'. Consequently we need to find and establish stability; this may work the body in unfamiliar ways and require considerable effort. Push the feet together!

There is also the question of what we need to release in order for this support to be cleanly transmitted. Sometimes people suggest that you simply have to 'let go' in an āsana – but this is an oversimplification: letting go of *unnecessary effort* allows you to find your real supports. This requires a commitment to the support that represents true *abhyāsa*. Simply 'letting go' can result in a posture becoming weak, insubstantial or impotent. Only when true support in a posture is found, can a radical letting go – *vairāgya* – arise. Now the posture can really touch us.

This is as much a mental attitude as a physical practice: can I let the posture really work on me whilst I remain open to its effect? We are inviting new feelings into the body, which can be challenging. Without such a step, āsana can simply reinforce pre-existing patterns, and this becomes a more subtle and enduring problem the more that we practise. We simply become more of who we already are! *Vairāgya* in āsana therefore allows us to be carried by a posture, opened up and profoundly touched by the experience. This is a letting go in order to turn *towards* the experience and its potential effects. In a sense, we 'get out of the way of ourselves'. In this way, even simple postures can restructure us – not in a negative sense, but by disrupting old physical patterns and opening up new possibilities. Instead of 'doing postures', we let them 'do us'.

The breath is the fundamental tool to find, clarify and

commit to our supports, and then to allow ourselves to be opened up and touched by the posture. Using the breath effectively is both an essential part of our method (*abhyāsa*) and, through its qualities, reflects the experience we hope to cultivate (*vairāgya*).[4]

When we breathe naturally in our everyday lives, the inhalation is the more active part of the breath, whereas the exhalation is a sort of 'rebound'; we relax as we breathe out and there is a 'letting go'. However, this can lead to a collapse on the exhalation. For example, when we stand in *samasthiti* with natural breathing, it is easy to experience a slight slumping with each exhalation, so that the space between the head and pelvis gradually reduces. Eventually, if unchecked, the cumulative effect of this exhaling will result in a rounded upper back and a slouched posture.

However, when we work with āsana and the breath in a more conscious and focused way, we can invert this relationship, so that the exhalation now becomes the more active aspect of the breath. Because the effort is applied more on the exhalation, we could say that this is the place of *abhyāsa*. One way of ensuring that this happens is to keep the head still as we breathe out, as if it is directly supported by the pelvis. This is done by tucking the chin in slightly as we exhale, and keeping the back of the neck lengthened, while lifting the sternum up towards the chin. This technique, called *jālandhara bandha* ('containing the nectar'[5]) is extremely effective for keeping the head steady as we exhale, and thereby avoiding a collapse of space between the head and the pelvis.

As well as maintaining the space between head and pelvis, *jālandhara bandha* also encourages a feeling of drawing the exhalation up from the lower abdomen. We apply effort to hold the head steady (but not so tightly that it creates neck tension) as we exhale. The effort of holding the head still as we exhale actually pulls the abdomen up and in, making it a firm platform from which to launch the subsequent inhalation. By maintaining and utilising this

4. See Chapter 9 for more extensive discussion on breath in āsana.

5. There are a number of ways of translating *jālandhara bandha*. In Haṭha Yoga, the head is considered to be the container of the 'nectar of immortality' (*amṛta*), a mythological fluid related to our longevity. This nectar is imagined as a fluid (*jāla*) that can be contained and stabilised (*dhara*) in this posture. This technique helps to keep the spine open and lengthened and is very important in both āsana and prāṇāyāma practices.

firmness of the abdomen as we breathe in, the inhalation becomes more relaxed and the body lengthens. We allow ourselves to be touched and opened by the inhalation. There is a feeling of letting be – *vairāgya* – as the breath opens a space deep within our axis and we grow taller.

To sum up: applying effort to the exhalation creates a stable base. We could say that the exhalation has something of the qualities of *abhyāsa*. The inhalation then enters and opens a clear space deep within us and we are touched. In this sense, the inhalation has something of *vairāgya*.[6]

These principles also apply to prāṇāyāma. Many elements in the practice of prāṇāyāma have a role in creating support and require us to engage with them carefully and diligently – this is *abhyāsa*. Examples of such elements include: the form of the posture for prāṇāyāma, the technique of prāṇāyāma, the length of the breath and structure of the practice. And once these are well established, *vairāgya* is very much related to how we give ourselves to the practice and how we allow it to restructure our experience. The practice opens a new space, allowing us to be more stable and more empowered, freer to make choices without compulsion.

In the same way, other aspects of our life can be informed by *abhyāsa* and *vairāgya*. Can we bring the qualities of *abhyāsa* to the disciplines and activities of our life so that we relate to them as useful supports? Our diet? Our lifestyle? Our relationships? And can we work with our attitudes so that we remain open to the experiences that they offer without becoming rigid, defensive or stuck? *Abhyāsa* gives us the support, direction and energy to keep moving forwards, and *vairāgya* gives us an openness to the richness of life without becoming stuck in the past or rigid about the future. This is freedom indeed, and a worthy aspiration for the practice of yoga.

6. This formulation of *abhyāsa* as linked to the exhalation and *vairāgya* as linked to the inhalation is consistent with the way we were taught and the way we teach. However, we acknowledge that other approaches to yoga may work in different ways with regard to the breath.

Chapter 6

व्याधिस्त्यानसंशयप्रमादालस्याविरति भ्रान्तिदर्शनालब्ध
भुमिकत्वानवस्थितत्वानि चित्तविक्षेपास्तेऽन्तरायाः।

Negotiating Obstacles

YS 1.30 vyādhi-styāna-saṃśaya-pramāda-ālasya-avirati-bhrāntidarśana-alabdhabhūmikatva-anavasthitatvāni citta-vikṣepāḥ te antarāyāḥ

Sickness, stagnation, doubt, carelessness, lethargy, indulgence, confusion of perspective, failure to progress and slipping back are interruptions on our journey towards a state of yoga

In our movement towards a state of *nirodha*, Patañjali recognises that there will inevitably be setbacks – sometimes brief, sometimes protracted. Because of the play of the *guṇa*, it is the very nature of our minds to fluctuate. Even if *sattva* is dominant and we are clear for a while, there is always the possibility of unexpected roadblocks on our journey. The word that Patañjali uses for these roadblocks is *antarāya,* which we could usefully translate as 'interruptions' or 'obstacles'. They come between us and our goal. They are 'internal' rather than external; that is to say, they originate in the mind rather than from outside. Unlike the *kleśa,* these interruptions are neither necessarily pervasive nor universal, instead they are seen as intermittent. There will be times in our lives when they manifest, other times when we are free of them. The *kleśa,* on the other hand, are an ongoing part of our lives. *Antarāya* are manifestations of imbalance, when *tamas* and/or *rajas* have become exaggerated and *sattva* has been eclipsed and obscured, resulting in disturbance and blockages in our systems.

At first glance, Patañjali's nine *antarāya* appear to be a random list. Although it is not traditional to do so, if we look at them in groups of three, a pattern emerges. The first group, comprising sickness (*vyādhi*), stagnation (*styāna*) and doubt (*saṃśaya*), arise from confusion with support. The second triad, comprising carelessness (*pramāda*), lassitude (*ālasya*) and indulgence (*avirati*) all indicate a misuse of energy. Finally, confusion of perspective (*bhrāntidarśana*), instability (*alabdha-bhūmikatva*) and slipping back (*anavasthitatvāni*), the third trio, are really about losing clear direction. These interruptions have the effect of becoming disturbances in our minds (*cittavikṣepāḥ*), and can result in certain symptoms in body, mind and breath which we shall explore in this chapter.

The first triad: Confusions with support

As is common in the Yoga Sūtra, Patañjali here presents us with a list – in this case, nine obstacles. We could see these as simply a list, with each having the potential to arise independently. However, we shall present them here as a sequential process whereby each has the potential to give birth to the next. Both perspectives have validity.

Vyādhi: Sickness

Although the word *vyādhi* is often translated as 'sickness', not all sickness is necessarily an obstacle; indeed, sometimes sickness can be transformative, a catalyst that propels us further along the path towards clarity and even emancipation. If we look more closely at the word we can unpick certain nuances which are not immediately obvious. *Vyādhi* comes from the root *dha,* meaning 'to place' or 'to support'. The prefix *vi* here means 'away from', thus *vyādhi* implies we are cut off from our support; we are displaced and out of touch with ourselves and, in this sense, we suffer from 'dis-ease'.

Healing – to make ourselves whole once more, to re-establish balance – is what is required, and the Indian medical system of āyurveda seeks to do just this. Two essential concepts in āyurveda are *prakṛti* and *vikṛti,* and understanding these helps us to understand *vyādhi.* In this context, *prakṛti* is our innate constitution, it is our state of balance and wellness – and each of us has his or her own unique *prakṛti.* Yet through lifestyle, diet and environmental factors, this state of balance can become disrupted and we move into what is called *vikṛti,* a state of imbalance. For many of us, for example, our heady electronic worlds cut us off from ourselves and we live in a fabricated palace of ideation as divorced from life as we are from the production of the food we consume from supermarkets. Although we often become habituated to our *vikṛti,* we feel very good when we return to our *prakṛti*; it is like coming home. Sitting quietly in nature, with little mental chatter, we can begin to realign, to breathe differently, to become more 'in tune' with ourselves. Āyurveda is about returning ourselves to ourselves when we have drifted away from our natural harmony and balance. There is no morality implied but rather an acknowledgement of our tendency to become divorced from our true support: our very Being. When we have 'returned to ourselves' we become *svastha,* firmly established (*stha*) in ourselves (*sva*). This is a profound state of mental and physical wellbeing and is the term used in āyurveda to mean 'health'.

Interestingly, the state of *samādhi* can be understood to be *vyādhi*'s polar opposite. *Samādhi* (it has the same root *dha*), meaning 'total integration', is the very state we seek to cultivate in our practice of yoga. Sometimes in modern yoga classes there can be an excessive emphasis on physical alignment, but in *samādhi* this alignment is far more profound and operates on all levels: here we are truly aligned with both ourselves and the reality of the Universe.

Styāna: Stagnation

Because *vyādhi* has taken us away from a state of balance, we try to rectify this situation by creating some stability, but often use 'false supports'. The next obstacle, *styāna* means 'stagnation' and comes from the root *stya* meaning 'to stiffen'. When we are removed from our essential support and in a state of *vyādhi,* we cling to what we might call 'false friends' – old habits and memories that give us a feeling of stability or certainty. However, this clinging creates a rigidity which fears change and can manifest as a loss of motivation, a feeling of complacency, or even simply a certain dogmatism and lack of openness. In *styāna,* we cling to the past and may become dull, fearful, or angry towards anyone or anything that challenges us.

For a support to function as a support rather than an addiction, we need to be free in our relationship to it. In *styāna* we become glued to our support. Interestingly, *vairāgya*[1] ('letting something be') and *styāna* can look similar – a certain indifference to, or rejection of, new possibilities. However, this would be to confuse the dullness

1. See Chapter 5.

and indifference that arises from the complacency of *styāna* with the openness of *vairāgya;* they are certainly not the same thing! *Styāna* shuts us down, with excessive clinging to ideas and viewpoints being one of its symptoms. In this sense *styāna,* which is often characterised by a rigid defensiveness, can be seen as the very opposite of *vairāgya.*

Saṃśaya: Doubt

Like so many words, the literal translation of *saṃśaya* as 'doubt' does not really do the term justice and can easily lead to misunderstanding and a rather crude view of the Yoga Sūtra. Sometimes, doubt is useful – we need some hesitation, some pondering, to counterbalance any tendency towards naivety or unthinking zeal – but this is not *saṃśaya*. Peter Hersnack said that *saṃśaya* "is that which consumes its own support".[2] It eats the very ground upon which we stand. Once the certainty of *styāna* becomes challenged, it becomes easy to lose all sense of stability and we lurch from one thing to another.

The root of the word is *śi*, meaning 'to rest'. Resting implies we take support and we can let go. *Sam,* like the English word 'sum', means 'bringing together'; thus, *saṃśaya* can be thought of as 'simultaneously resting in two places'. This is problematic. In order for us to move in any direction, we need to be secure in our support. When we are secure in our support, a direction becomes clearer – and even if we are not *completely* clear about where we are moving towards (direction), we need to know where we are moving from (support). Then, sometimes slowly, a direction may reveal itself.

If we understand *saṃśaya* as 'taking support from two different places simultaneously', we can see how this has the potential to confuse the direction immensely. A direction cannot become clear when we are jumping (physically or mentally) between two different 'givens', and this is how *saṃśaya* consumes its support; it erodes the baseline from which we move.

2. Personal communication.

The confusion and doubt of *saṃśaya* is the state of the hero Arjuna at the beginning of the *Bhagavad Gītā*. Arjuna is about to go to war, and yet on the eve of the battle he falls into despair and his thoughts become confused and conflicted. His duty as a warrior is to fight – and yet he finds himself facing his own family and teachers. Should he fight for a just cause or should he lay down his arms and be killed? The great warrior is reduced to a feeble state; his doubts make him barely able to lift his bow, his body trembles and he is consumed by great mental anguish. Doubt is often crippling, and its resolution is sometimes complex – Arjuna's perspective is carefully realigned by his teacher, Kṛṣṇa, over the rest of the text. This is a journey involving harsh words, gentle coaxing, analogies, direct teachings, praise and admonishments.

For us to move forward, we need the opposite of *saṃśaya*: confidence and trust. In Sanskrit, this is known as *śraddhā*. All healing requires *śraddhā*; it enables us to take some risks, to make mistakes and to persevere. Whenever we learn something new, and persevere with that learning as we take another tentative footstep forward, we have *śraddhā*. It is the fuel that powers us out of our habitual orbits and into the unknown – although we all have our setbacks and our challenges, *śraddhā* keeps us learning and evolving.

The second triad: Misuse of energy

This second triad concerns the consequences of misusing our energy. When we have good support in place, our energy can be directed and take us far. However, when we use our energy *as* the support, it burns up – and we eventually burn out. Our energy is not topped up and increasingly we need to rely on 'false supports'.

Pramāda: Carelessness

When we have plenty of time, money or energy, or we are suffering from extreme doubt, we can become indulgent and careless. Launching ourselves into a new endeavour or experience can be a way of overcoming indecision, but we can misspend or overspend without necessarily noticing or caring. The root of *pramāda* is *mad*, which means 'intoxicated' or 'drunk'. In such a state, it is easy to squander our assets and live on borrowed or dwindling resources. We become increasingly hasty and reckless and our obsession encourages us to neglect our other responsibilities. But this way of living has consequences. If we survive on borrowed energy, we still have to repay the energetic debt – and often with considerable interest.

Pramāda is about being intoxicated in some form. This might be physical but, equally, we can be impatient for an outcome, overly hasty or neglectful. Sometimes, this very feeling of intoxication becomes a sort of false support: we get habituated and then addicted to 'the buzz'. Of course, this means we are not living in the moment. Instead we are running on adrenalin and are too 'wired' to take time, to take notice, to breathe.

Ālasya: Lethargy

This is the hangover – we have used up our energy and now we are 'spent'. The root *as* means 'to shine'. The state of *ālasya* is a state of dullness: we feel lacklustre, idle and exhausted. Āyurveda describes *ojas* as the final product of good digestion. *Ojas* is a substance that confers immunity, good digestion and general health. In one who has good *ojas* there is a glow, a natural brightness in the eyes and a radiant quality to the skin, and a sweetness in their nature. However, when we misuse our energy, abusing our lifestyle and diet, the production of *ojas* is severely compromised and we experience the state of *ālasya*. Our skin and eyes lose their lustre, we look tired and dull, and we lack enthusiasm, fortitude and happiness.

Avirati: Indulgence

When one is feeling dull, a common, if not wise solution, is indulgence. *Avirati* completes this three-part cycle –

from *pramāda,* (intoxication, in whatever form) to *ālasya* (depletion and lethargy), and finally to *avirati,* stimulation and indulgence to get going again. *Avirati* refers to this over-indulgence or intemperance. When our supports are totally external, we often find the need for stronger and stronger stimuli to motivate us. The root of the word is *ram,* meaning the 'enjoyment of pleasure'. The prefix *vi* means 'against' and '*a*' makes this a double negative. Thus, *avirati* is 'not stopping ourselves indulging'; it is the desire to (over)feed our senses. When we are out of touch with ourselves and lacking sensitivity, we need gross stimulation just to feel alive – and the process is addictive.

The third triad: Losing clear direction

The third triad explores how our direction can become confused, unstable or elusive, and out of our reach.

Bhrāntidarśana: Confusion of perspective

The word *bhrānti* means 'wandering off' or 'wavering' and in this context it means both false and unstable. *Darśana* is a 'viewpoint' – so *bhrāntidarśana* is a skewed perspective, something which is 'a bit off'. Of course, this can happen at any time, but if we see this as a cyclical process which is preceded by the first six *antarāya,* it is not surprising that our understanding is muddled because our energies have become depleted from *ālasya* and have been artificially stimulated (*avirati*) so that *rajas* predominates: a 'perfect storm' for confusion.

Alabdhabhūmikatva: Failure to progress

To reach a goal is *labdha,* thus *alabdha* is for that goal to remain unfulfilled. This is often because of a refusal to take a vital step, for whatever reason. For example, there may be a lack of trust or self-confidence, or a reluctance to move out of our comfort zone. There may also be inadequate preparation. *Bhūmi* is 'ground', and *bhūmikatva* means 'having the qualities of the ground'. If the ground has not been well prepared, it cannot provide us with the optimum support for reaching our goals. This is really about proper *vinyāsa krama* – the intelligent steps we make in our chosen direction. Of course, if the steps are muddled or problematic, we are much more likely to fail. Here, our direction is lost. Patañjali reiterates this point in YS 3.6, *tasya bhūmiṣu viniyogaḥ*: yoga should evolve in stages (*bhūmi*).[3]

The term *bhūmi* also relates to our physical nature, our 'earth', our embodied being. It is not uncommon for us to know something intellectually but for it to stay just that – knowledge that remains at the level of theory. In YS 1.3, Patañjali describes a state of embodied Being (*draṣṭuḥ avasthānam*), and for yoga to really mean something, our insights and our practices must inform and slowly transform our very being in the world. This takes time to evolve, and a slow and gradual process of transformation is required in order to avoid *alabdhabhūmikatva*. It is not uncommon to give up prematurely, to somehow sabotage our success, even if our preparations have been sound. It is important to remember that yoga is a slow burn that requires diligence, patience and faith. Embodiment takes time.

Anavasthitatvāni: Slipping back

In the middle of this rather daunting word is *sthiti*, a word we know well which means 'stability'. In *anavasthitatvāni*, the quality of stability eludes us and even if we reach a goal, we cannot maintain it and we slide back. As we saw in the previous chapter, *yoga-kṣema* is an important principle here: it means the ability to maintain where we have reached. Often people make good progress at the beginning of their yoga career and are struck by revelations and new experiences. But the honeymoon period ends, and eventually disillusionment may set in. It's worth repeating: yoga is a long journey. There will be times when circumstances are such that we need to simply tread water, to wait until conditions are better for progress. The journey is not a straight line and there will

3. See Chapter 3.

be many plateaus along the way. Just as there are fallow times and growth spurts in the life of a plant, so it is in our practice. Sometimes we are ill, or our family situation is such that practice needs to be 'put on the back burner'. And sometimes this can be for years! At times it would be easy to simply give up, but the important teaching here is that maintaining some link, keeping the flame alight so that it can grow when circumstances are more conducive, is essential.

The symptoms of *antarāya*

YS 1.31 duḥkha-daurmanasya-aṅgamejayatva-śvāsa-praśvāsa vikṣepa-sahabhuvaḥ

Emotional distress, negative thinking, unsteadiness in the body and disturbed breathing patterns arise with these disturbances of mind (antarāya)

The obstacles presented in YS 1.30 manifest through the channels described in YS 1.31. These are the symptoms of our yoga journey having been interrupted. As we have seen, classical Indian philosophy sees no body–mind split, because both body and mind are part of *prakṛti*. We might go as far as to say that the body is the grossest manifestation of the mind; our bodies reveal something of the mind. This is obvious when we consider posture and expression, when our bodies involuntarily communicate something of our mental attitude.

In the same way, our breathing is intimately related to our state of mind, and of course the health of our body. Here Patañjali states that *antarāya* gives rise to emotional, cognitive, physical or respiratory symptoms. We may feel distressed and restricted (*duḥkha*); we may be plagued by negative thoughts (*daurmanasya*); we may find our bodies shaky and unstable (*aṅgamejayatva*); and finally our breathing may be short, erratic or compromised (*śvāsa-praśvāsa*).

The first symptom, *duḥkha*, is an experience of restriction. Physically, this might be a feeling of tightness in the chest or heart, but it is primarily an emotional experience, cutting us off from our ability to feel joy. The second symptom, *daurmanasya,* literally means 'bad mind'. Here our thinking is muddled and we see the world through a fog of gloom which poisons our perceptions. When we experience disturbance at the physical level, we may become unsteady or start to tremble: this is called *aṅgamejayatva,* the third symptom. Finally, *śvāsa-praśvāsa* is a disturbance in our breathing: we may breathe rapidly or erratically and we may inadvertently hold our breath or gasp. These are symptoms of disruption on the energetic level and this disturbance may also manifest in our pulse.[4] Of course, how we feel may affect how we breathe, how we think or how we hold ourselves; they are all inter-related. But often one channel is more obvious and is the driver of the others.

Nine solutions to *antarāya*

Patañjali presents nine solutions to the problems arising from *antarāya*. In some ways, the suggested practices in the first chapter of the Yoga Sūtra are little hints, and many of them are elaborated in considerably more detail both in the second chapter, where Patañjali discusses *yama* and *prāṇāyāma*, and also in the third chapter where various possibilities are presented as objects for contemplation. These include friendliness (YS 3.23), aspects of our energetic system (YS 3.39–48), the light of perfected Beings (YS 3.32) and many aspects of the universe, including the sun, moon, and pole star (YS 3.26–3.28), each of which has an internal corollary in our own systems. Fundamental to all of the practices is the reduction of excessive *tamas* and *rajas*, and the cultivation of *sattva guṇa*. We cannot emphasise this enough: when *tamas* and *rajas* are able to fulfil their positive functions, *tamas* provides support, *rajas* give energy to the direction, and *sattva,* the feeling of spaciousness, increases. But when they are in excess, *tamas* and *rajas* are simply impediments.

Below, we look at sūtras YS1.29, and then 1.32–39 in more depth where Patañjali suggests some ways to reduce the effects of *antarāya*. Note that he is not prescriptive, but rather offers a

4. A disturbance in the breath is really a disturbance of our *prāṇa*, and from an āyurvedic perspective, this can be felt in our pulse.

number of alternative practical solutions (this is indicated by his use of the word '*vā*' which means 'or').

YS 1.29 tataḥ pratyak-cetanā adhigamaḥ api-antarāya-abhāvaśca

(From a devotional attitude) we move inwards and obstacles do not arise

Before presenting the *antarāya*, Patañjali makes some interesting observations about the cultivation of a devotional attitude (*īśvara praṇidhāna*).[5] First of all, in YS 1.23 he says that this is an optional path: he neither demands it, nor does he give form to *īśvara* (sometimes translated as God, but here we can say 'The Highest Power'). *Īśvara* is simply the object of devotion. He goes on to say in YS 1.29 that this practice will result in two things: a flowering of inner awareness (*pratyak-cetanā*) and also that there will be a lack of fertile soil for obstacles to grow in (*antarāya abhāva*). Of course, this is not to say that anyone with faith will remain free of sickness, doubts, indulgence, confusion and the rest. However, arising from *īśvara praṇidhāna* is a profound feeling of connection, of 'being held', and this feeling releases us from a mindset which is the breeding ground for *rajas* and *tamas*. At its purest, *īśvara praṇidhāna* promotes *sattva*;[6] we are able to move on and thereby remain relatively light, and free of *antarāya*.

YS 1.32 tat pratiṣedha-artham eka-tattva-abhyāsaḥ

Focus on one thing at a time

The cultivation of a stable awareness is perhaps the single most important practice in Patañjali's yoga, and focusing on one essential principle (*eka-tattva*) at a time is paramount. It is both the means of refining one's awareness and also the fruit of the practice: it requires *sattva*, spaciousness, to be supported and stabilised by *tamas* and

5. See Chapter 16.

6. Confused *īśvara praṇidhāna* can promote fanaticism, sectarianism and intolerance – all hallmarks of excessive *rajas* and *tamas*.

given energy and direction by *rajas*. In such conditions, our ability to stay with our chosen focus is immense. However, the antithesis of this state is multi-tasking, 'channel-hopping' as it were, from one thing to another. This is the normal state of affairs and is exacerbated by digital media and modern lifestyles. Unfortunately, the consequence of such flitting is more than simply instability, agitation and the inability to focus. A stable mind is also a happy mind, while an unstable mind is distressed. With the *guṇa* out of balance, an unstable mind is a natural breeding ground for *antarāya*. We cannot emphasise enough: yoga is a slow process and it takes patience, commitment and perseverance – but like a ripening fruit, it has a sweet taste. There are many possible practices in yoga and it is easy to feel overwhelmed or distracted with the multitude of possibilities. This sūtra offers very simple and sound advice: come back to one important principle or focus, and then stay with it.

YS 1.33 maitrī-karuṇā muditā-upekṣāṇām sukha-duḥkha-puṇya-apuṇya-viṣayāṇām bhāvanātaḥ citta prasādanam

Cultivating friendliness, compassion, happiness and equanimity to those who are happy, unhappy, virtuous or not virtuous will clear the mind

We could easily write a whole chapter just on this sūtra, since it contains such important advice. Indeed, Patañjali's teachings here are a direct echo of those of the Buddha whose 'four virtues' (known as the *brahmavihāra*) are the cornerstone of Buddhist practice and ethics. Patañjali emphasises that we are not alone; we exist as part of different networks and how we act within these networks will radically influence our state of mind. The whole approach to relationships is considerably expanded in YS 2.30–2.39,[7] but Patañjali succinctly gives us four attitudes to cultivate in four different arenas. Towards the happy

7. See Chapter 11.

(*sukha*), we can be friendly (*maitrī*); towards the unhappy (*duḥkha*) we can be compassionate (*karuṇā*); towards the virtuous (*puṇya*) we can display goodwill (*muditā*); and towards those who are behaving unethically (*apuṇya*) we may show some equanimity (*upekṣāṇām*). By cultivating these qualities (*bhāvanātaḥ*) the mind (*citta*) becomes clear (*prasādanam*).

This sūtra highlights the importance of yoga practice *off* the mat – it needs to inform our relationships and our conduct, lest the focus we cultivate on our mat is dissipated by our interactions and our being in the world. The stable and spacious quality of *sattva* can easily be unsettled or obscured by disdain, contempt, jealousy or hatred.

YS 1.34 pracchardana-vidhāraṇābhyāṃ vā prāṇasya

Or explore your exhalation and the pause after it

Although Patañjali goes on in YS 2.49–53 to elaborate on his teaching of prāṇāyāma in considerable detail, here he is introducing the idea that breathing practices, in particular the exhalation and subsequent pause, are key factors in stabilising the mind and aiding the health of the body. The exhalation and subsequent pause[8] are intimately linked to the energy of *apāna vāyu* whose function is to 'clear out', cleanse and help us move on. These aspects of the breath most directly address our blockages, be they physical, mental or emotional, and it is therefore unsurprising that Patañjali emphasises their practice as a way to reduce *antarāya*.

YS 1.35 viṣaya-vatī vā pravṛttir utpannā manasaḥ sthiti-nibandhinī

Or consider sense objects

Although some of the traditional commentators understand this sūtra to refer to quite esoteric experiences which

8. See Chapter 10 for further discussion.

transcend ordinary sensations,[9] we can usefully see this sūtra to apply to readily accessible experiences. Very simply: stability of mind arises from carefully attending to our sense perceptions. Becoming overwhelmed by obstacles and interruptions moves us away from our true supports and we become increasingly cut off and isolated. It is the opposite of *svastha,* where we are grounded in ourselves and feel embodied. One of the most direct portals to come back to the present moment is to focus (*pravṛtti*) on the objects of the senses (*viṣaya-vatī*), and this focusing brings a profound steadiness (*sthiti nibandhinī*) to the mind (*manas*). Here Patañjali uses the term *manas* to discuss the mind rather than *citta*, because *manas* is that part of the mind most intimately linked to the senses. This is the deliberate practice of cultivating presence by focusing on the now – it, quite literally, 'brings us back to our senses'.[10] This practice has become hugely popular through the contemporary practice of mindfulness which is used therapeutically in many situations – for example, as stress-reduction, anger management and for depression.

YS 1.36 viśokā vā jyotiṣmatī

Or (focus on) a pure light which is free from all pain and suffering

As with the previous sūtra, this has been interpreted by some of the traditional commentators in quite an obscure manner. Vyāsa alludes to the subtle body and esoteric anatomy, including visions of the sun, moon, planets and precious gems arising from focus on the heart. Whilst these may be quite valid, we can think of this sūtra more simply in terms of *guṇa*: *jyotiṣmatī* means 'luminous' and 'full of light' and is synonymous with *sattva*. One of the qualities of *sattva* is that it is joyous and therefore free from pain and suffering (*viśokā*). There is a part of us that remains untouched by our suffering and pain. By cultivating *sattva guṇa* and focusing on the heart (as Vyāsa says), we can access that transcendental

9. Vyāsa discusses how (amongst other points of focus), concentration on the tip of the nose results in a subtle sense of smell, the tip of the tongue gives a subtle sense of taste and even focus on the palette can alter our perception of colour.

10. For a detailed discussion on the role of the senses see Chapter 14.

aspect of ourselves to help navigate our way through or around *antarāya*.

YS 1.37 vīta-rāga-viṣayaṃ vā cittam

Or (focus on) someone who embodies a mastery of their passions and desires

We all have the potential to be moved and inspired by, for example, our family and friends, fictional characters in novels or films, or those who have overcome adversity and gone on to achieve something remarkable. Heroes and heroines in the classical myths of all cultures inspire us to transcend our limits and push our boundaries. Although it is easy to become jaded and cynical – we love to knock our heroes off their pedestals – it is also important to acknowledge the many people who have shown us something of value. A picture, memory or idea of someone special can be such a touchstone, helping us move past our blockages with stability and clarity of mind. Here Patañjali suggests that we can find such inspiration by focusing on someone who embodies the qualities of equanimity and who is not pulled by their passions and desires (*vīta-rāga*).

YS 1.38 svapna-nidrā jñāna-ālambanaṃ vā

Or explore your dreams and the state of dreamless sleep

The exploration of both dreams (*svapna*) and dreamless sleep (*nidrā*) is a common theme in classical Indian thought, and they have been the subject of much speculation. In some of the Upaniṣads, for example, the *Māṇḍūkya Upaniṣad*, dreams, dreamless sleep and the waking state of ordinary consciousness are contrasted to the consciousness of one who has achieved liberation (*mokṣa*). Dreams, dreamless sleep and waking consciousness are all variable because they fluctuate with the *guṇa*, and they are all states that can be observed or experienced. This is in direct contrast to that of *cit* or *puruṣa*, whose state cannot be observed and whose awareness remains constant because it is unaffected by *guṇa*. *Puruṣa* is that which observes the other states.

Even though there are similarities between dreaming, dreamless sleep and waking consciousness, dreamless sleep is given a special significance because it is a state of *citta vṛtti nirodha*, albeit an unconscious and therefore a 'tamasic' one. Dreamless sleep is, as we know, a vital part of maintaining our wellbeing and without it we quickly succumb to various health problems, both physical and mental. It helps us to 'wipe our systems clean' and refreshes us for the next day. In this sense, it has some similarities to various practices from yoga, especially the deep meditative state of *samādhi*.

From ancient tribal cultures through to modern psychotherapy, dreams are given special significance – they may be prophetic or simply shine a light on some aspect of our lives. They can be like mirrors to our waking states, reflecting what is unconscious and thereby allowing us, at least to some extent, to become transparent to ourselves. Many stories from religious traditions hinge on a dream or a vision – from Noah's Ark and Mary's immaculate conception in the Bible to the transmission of lost texts to Krishnamacharya[11] in the yoga tradition. Sometimes they can be disturbing, although what Patañjali suggests here is that the meanings and insights they offer (*jñāna*) may reveal a path around the blockages caused by *antarāya* and towards a place of stability and inspiration.

YS 1.39 yathā-abhimata dhyānād-vā

Or focus on anything that brings steadiness

This sūtra reveals the pragmatism and openness of Patañjali's teachings. As we have seen, he does not demand adherence to a particular religious tradition, to a particular path or to a particular doctrine. Desikachar often pointed out that yoga (and by that he meant yoga grounded in the Yoga Sūtra) should make a Christian a better Christian, a Muslim a better Muslim and an atheist a better atheist. These teachings are

11. Krishnamacharya is said to have received the full text of the *Yoga Rahasya* from his ancestor Nāthamuni in a dream (see p. 39).

about promoting healthier, happier and clearer lives and anything that is agreeable (*abhimata*) can become an object of our meditation (*dhyāna*) and help us to become steady. It is easier for our minds to focus on something agreeable or interesting, and it is this very process of focusing which, as we have seen, brings both steadiness to the mind and relief from disturbing thoughts. If, for example, drawing is your passion, that can help you to stabilise. Indeed, any focus can act like an anchor, steadying us in a sea of conflicting forces.

Sādhana: Variations and modifications

In many modern yoga classes, we often find students struggling to emulate their teacher, or an idea of what the posture should look like. How far should the feet be apart? Should my hand face forward or backwards? A common question from students is "what is the classical form?" But as Mark Singleton points out in *Yoga Body*,[12] one of the unexpected consequences of the advent of photography was exactly this development of standard and ideal forms in āsana. It is far more difficult to define a 'classical' form of āsana by looking at the earlier illustrations and paintings.

Likewise, the descriptions of āsana in classical texts such as the *Haṭha Yoga Pradīpikā* (HYP) are rather vague and, without a teacher, it is difficult to know how to practise. For example, the HYP describes the bow posture (*dhanurāsana*) thus:

> "Having caught the toes of the foot with both hands and carried them to the ears by drawing the body like a bow, it becomes *dhanurāsana*" (HYP 1.27).[13]

A tall order for anyone to follow!

Before āsana were photographed, all teachers could work with was the actual person in front of them; there was no external blueprint to aspire to. Indeed, one of the hallmarks of both āyurveda and yoga is that we

12. Singleton, op. cit.

13. The *Haṭhayogapradīpikā* of Svātmārāma, The Adyar Library and Research Centre, Madras, 1972.

are all individual: what is right for one person may be inappropriate for another. There is no 'one-size-fits-all' approach to Indian spirituality.

Patañjali is very open about his solutions to *antarāya*: you could try *this*, or if that doesn't work – how about *that*? Hence all those 'or's in the sūtras above. Similarly, in the *Bhagavad Gītā*, Kṛṣṇa extols the virtue of many different paths to yoga, many different practices. He acknowledges that different people, with differing potentials, interests and circumstances, will need different approaches to spirituality. It was this very principle that first attracted us to the work of Desikachar. As we saw in Chapter 3, postures (indeed, yoga itself) should be adapted to the individual, rather than the other way around. The important point in relation to āsana is to understand the principles of form and function: what are we trying to achieve in this posture, and how can we best adapt the form to respect that goal? We have already discussed the concept of *rakṣana*[14] and we can appreciate that such an approach protects both the *function* of the posture and the practitioner. This is usually done by adapting or modifying the āsana. For example, bending the knees and side-sweeping the arms in *uttānāsana* closes the hips and reduces loading in the back (fig 6.1).

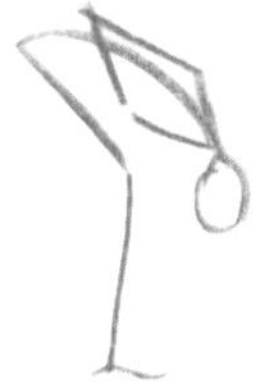

fig 6.1

Modifications bring us *towards* a posture. For many, trying to achieve the 'final form' of a posture without making certain changes, could lead to little benefit at best and serious injury at worst. Āsana modifications are an extremely effective tool in negotiating obstacles we may

14. See Chapter 3.

face in our practice. In other words, just because we can't touch our toes does not mean we cannot practise āsana! As Krishnamacharya is reported to have said, "where there is breath, there is hope."

Variations, on the other hand, are usually performed in order to add interest, or work with a specific idea. Variations take us *away* from the usual function of a posture by introducing a new element which is not essential to the posture. In this case, we are adapting the form of the āsana in order to experience a new sensation.

Most variations involve placing the limbs into unusual positions. There are many arm variations which can be applied to a whole range of postures. We may place the arms in a reverse prayer position, place the hands on the shoulder blades, or cross the hands behind our head. We may also put the arms in a '*gomukha*' position, linking hands behind the back with one elbow up and one elbow down.

Similarly, we can place the legs into a variety of positions in āsana that may otherwise require the legs to be straight or symmetrical. For example, we may wish to work with lotus posture and so we can add the half-lotus leg position to other seated postures as a way of preparing the legs, hips and knees (*ardha padma paścimatānāsana*, fig 6.2).

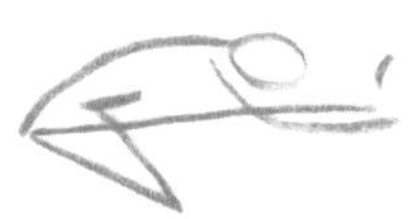

fig 6.2

Although slightly less common, another way of creating variation in āsana is by changing the alignment of the spine. When the spine is in neutral or in flexion, we can introduce a twist (*parivṛtti*) to intensify the posture and bring in a new experience, for example, in *parivṛtti tāḍāsana* (fig 6.3).

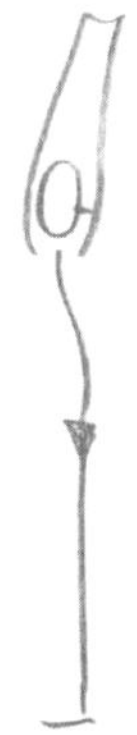

fig 6.3

Variations can help to push our practice and deepen our involvement at both the physical and psychological level. Variations can also be very helpful in overcoming obstacles, for example, when we become stale and our practice lacks interest. They are there to help us see something from a different angle, to explore new avenues and keep us enthused and fresh.

Chapter 7

प्रकाशक्रियास्थितिशीलं भूतेन्द्रियात्मकं
भोगापवर्गार्थं दृश्यम् ।

The Nature of Things

YS 2.18 prakāśa-kriyā-sthiti-śīlaṃ bhūta-indriya-ātmakaṃ bhoga-apavargārthaṃ dṛśyaṃ

Luminosity (prakāśa), activity (kriyā) and stability (sthiti) are the essential qualities (śīla) that make up the entire observable world (dṛśya). They are also the nature (ātmaka) of our own senses (indriya), and indeed of all of our bodies and the external world. Everything that exists is there to be experienced (bhoga) – and has the potential either to further enmesh us, or to set us free (apavarga)

This extremely important sūtra synthesises the heart of the philosophy of Sāṃkhya and indeed of yoga. It explains the nature of the material world, and describes how its characteristics run right through our subjective senses and the objective world that we perceive. It also explains that the phenomenal world has two primary purposes, and that for most of us, there is an order to them.

The material world is simply *prakṛti* – everything of which we can be aware. It is made up of three strands; *prakāśa* (light), *kriyā* (movement) and *sthiti* (stability). These are clever synonyms for *sattva*, *rajas* and *tamas.* One of *sattva's* qualities is *prakāśa*, it is luminous. The very nature of *rajas* is *kriyā*, activity. And *tamas* can be understood as inertia, resistance and thus stability, *sthiti.* These three *guṇa* permeate our senses (called *indriya* in the Yoga Sūtra), and our minds, and also the very elements (*bhūta*) which we perceive in the external world (including our physical bodies). Interestingly, and crucially, our senses, our minds and the world which we perceive are described as *dṛśya* – 'seen'. Our senses and minds can be 'seen' because we can step back and be aware of their operation. Perhaps they are dull, perhaps acute – but we can observe how they change and thus they are included as part of *prakṛti*, the objective world of phenomena.

Finally, this sūtra ends with an extremely arresting statement: that the purpose (*artha*) of this world of phenomena is twofold. It is there for us to experience (*bhoga*), and then to transcend (*apavarga*). In other words, experiences are the very means to liberation and freedom. This liberation is called *apavarga*. It's worth noting that not all *bhoga* leads us to *apavarga* – indeed much *bhoga* will take us in exactly the wrong direction! What is important here is that only through skilfully lived experience does emancipation arise.[1]

1. The relationship between *bhoga* and *apavarga* has been the subject of much debate in the Indian spiritual tradition. Some extreme renunciate traditions shun *bhoga* and focus exclusively on *apavarga*, whilst others proclaim the necessity of *bhoga* as the means.

Incarnation

It is utterly extraordinary that we are alive. According to one Buddhist parable, the chances of being born a human are similar to a turtle, who swims up from the depths of the ocean once in a thousand years, putting its head through a single ring floating on the surface of the water. A man produces billions of sperm during his lifetime; just think how incredible it is that of all those, only one yoked with one of your mother's (many thousands of) eggs and... became *you*. It's worth reminding ourselves just how unlikely – and how precious – our existence truly is.

The ancient Indian philosophers also emphasised that being born into the human realm is a particular blessing because we are born with just the right amount of insight. Being born into the realms of animals means existing 'as animals': living primarily by instinct and without spiritual insight. In this realm, the primary drives are food, pleasure, avoidance of danger and so on, and this level is dominated by *rajas* and *tamas*. (It could easily be argued that some people live only in this realm). At the other end of the spectrum is living in the realms of the Gods, the so-called *devaloka*. According to mythology, this is dominated by *sattva,* it is a place of beauty and enjoyment and clarity. But – and it's an important 'but' – there is too little suffering to make us want to explore the true nature of things; we are too cosy. Only in the human realm is there sufficient clarity *and* suffering: we are in the 'Goldilocks orbit' – neither so far away that we have no insight nor so comfortable that there is no need to resolve our confusions and difficulties.

Puruṣa

Intuitively, we distinguish between inside and outside with our skin – everything internal to the skin is 'us' and everything external is 'other'. But as we have seen, yoga demarcates this boundary in another way: what is 'internal' is the witness (*puruṣa*) and everything else is 'external' – it is the 'witnessed'. What we normally think of as internal to our bodies (our lungs expanding, our heartbeat, our muscles working) can be observed and, from the point of view of yoga, is actually external. It forms part of *dṛśya*, the Seen.

How do we understand that which is 'internal'? Yoga suggests that by contrast to *prakṛti*,[2] there is an essence which does not change: this is called *puruṣa*. *Puruṣa* is very difficult to talk about, however, because by naming it, we describe it, and thereby turn it into 'a thing'. We give it qualities, form and substance: we treat it as *prakṛti*. Yet *puruṣa* has no form, no place, no time. It is the subject, rather than the object, of investigation. Rather poetically, Peter Hersnack once described *puruṣa* as "always the same, but always fresh."[3]

The boundary between 'inside' and 'outside' is thus not the skin, but the distinction between *puruṣa* and *prakṛti* – terms for which Patañjali uses many synonyms throughout the Yoga Sūtra. This is as much a problem of language as one of perception: without clothing 'it'[4] in words, we would have no way of talking about *puruṣa*. Patañjali's numerous terms help to give us various perspectives on *puruṣa*:

- *cit* – awareness (YS 4.22 and 4.34)
- *draṣṭṛ* – the Seer (YS 1.3, 2.17, 2.20 and 4.23)
- *ātman* – the essence (YS 2.5, 2.21, 2.41 and 4.25)
- *puruṣa* – person, the dweller in the city (YS 1.16, 1.24, 3.35, 3.49, 3.55, 4.18 and 4.34)

Each of these terms gives us a slightly different angle on the concept of *puruṣa*. It is awareness (*cit*) that receives information and content from our minds in the form of memories, the imagination or information from our senses. However, this awareness is separate from, and fundamentally untouched by, that content. Similarly, it is the Seer (*draṣṭṛ*) who receives all sensory information – and not just visual, but all the smells, tastes, feelings and sounds from the external world. If we lose a limb, of course we will feel differently about who we are to an extent, but we may

2. *Dṛśyaṃ* and *prakṛti* are interchangeable names for Nature.

3. Personal communication. The reason that it is 'always the same' is because it is out of time; time is a product of *prakṛti*. Time is about change: where there is no change, there is no time.

4. Even calling *puruṣa* 'it' is problematic, because we run the risk of 'nounifying' – turning it into a 'thing'.

lose limbs, have organs transplanted, hips replaced and still feel, in some ways, like 'ourselves'. The *ātman* – sometimes translated as the 'soul' – refers to that which remains when all the changing forms that constitute our identity have been taken away. In the Yoga Sūtra, this essence is construed as having no qualities. Finally, we could conceive of the body/mind complex rather like a city or a palace (*pura*) whose 'inhabitant' is *puruṣa* – the dweller in the city.

One simple and practical way to get something of the flavour of *puruṣa's* presence is to borrow a concept from Vedānta[5] philosophy: that of *sat* (being), *cit* (awareness) and *ānanda* (bliss). In Vedānta, the very ground of being, the basis of all, is called *Brahman* and its qualities are described as *sat-cit-ānanda*. With this as our touchstone, we can intuit the presence of *puruṣa*. At the end of a practice, sitting or standing quietly, ask yourself: is there presence (*sat*)? Is there awareness and sensitivity (*cit*)? Is there joy, bliss (*ānanda*)? These can be taken as the signs, the markings, of the presence of *puruṣa*.

Although we have taken the liberty of discussing the various ways Patañjali has given form to *puruṣa*, we must always remember that, ultimately, *puruṣa* is *nirguṇa* (without qualities), whilst *prakṛti* is *saguṇa* (with qualities).

Prakṛti and *Guṇa*

The classical Indian tradition understands *prakṛti* (or *dṛśya,* the observable world) to be comprised of three fundamental forces: the three *guṇa* – *sattva, rajas* and *tamas.* It includes our bodies, and even our minds, thoughts, memories, feelings and emotions. Our thoughts and feelings are simply 'stuff' – they are more subtle (less stable and tangible) than our legs and arms, but all 'stuff' is subject to change – it grows, moves and decays. Stuff is subject to *guṇa*. It has qualities and is therefore describable. It gets recycled and remoulded into other stuff; thoughts evolve into other thoughts and even into physical realities (a

5. Vedānta is another of India's classical philosophies arising from the Veda. Although the most well known of India's classical philosophical systems, in some ways it is quite different from the classical yoga tradition. However, there are also many shared ideas and concepts between the two systems and an understanding of yoga is certainly very helpful as a basis for understanding Vedānta.

thought can mould an expression or a posture); likewise, the material of our bodies is recycled into other bodies. Yoga makes no distinction between mind and body – both are simply aspects of *prakṛti*. There is nothing stable or eternal about our identities or our thoughts; these will change just as the cells of our bodies will be replaced. As we have seen, all of this can, in some sense, be thought of as 'external', because it can be observed.

It is worth taking time to really understand the three *guṇa* because they lie at the heart of traditional Indian philosophy. There are a number of common misunderstandings in the contemporary yoga world about the *guṇa* and their relationships with each other. Many people talk of trying to 'balance' the *guṇa,* as if they could all come into a sort of equilibrium and stay there. Often people see *tamas* and *rajas* as undesirable, not understanding that their presence is essential and that they both have positive roles to play in the dance of life. Exploring how the *guṇa* are presented in the *Sāṃkhya Kārikā* (SK) gives us great insight into their meaning and use in the Yoga Sūtra. In SK 12 and 13, their purpose, their interactions with one another, and their essential characteristics are explained with masterly brevity and precision.

In SK 12, the effect of the three *guṇa* on our minds is presented. The text states that the effect of *sattva* is joy (*prīti*), that of *rajas* is pain (*aprīti*), and finally *tamas* brings a feeling of despair (*viṣāda*). The joy of *sattva* does not necessarily mean an ecstatic, loud or external joy; it is more a peaceful beatitude, a feeling of being blessed. The experience of *rajas* is pain – wherever there is pain there is *rajas*. *Rajas* provokes movement, and there is nothing to make us move as quickly as the experience of pain. It stimulates. The effect of *tamas* is despair: a giving up and an impotent resignation. *Tamas* is there to block – it may block movement, feeling, understanding or initiative.

Although, put like this, the effects of *rajas* and *tamas* seem undesirable, they serve an important purpose.

SK 12 goes on to explain that while *sattva* is there to bring illumination (*prakāśa*), *rajas* brings movement (*pravṛtti*) and *tamas* restraint (*niyama*). None of these are inherently good or bad: they simply are. Without the movement of *rajas* or the restraint of *tamas* there would be no time, no growth and no boundaries. Once the dance of the *guṇa* has started, it is really impossible to bring them into balance, because they are in constant dynamic relationship with one another, and their presence and interactions bring forth the world of form.

SK 12 describes their interactions with one another in four ways; we can further subdivide this into two pairs. In the first, one *guṇa* dominates (*abhibhava vṛtti*), and another supports (*āśraya vṛtti*). There will always be a dominant *guṇa* in any situation, but how that dominant *guṇa* manifests will be dependent on how it is supported. For example, when *rajas* is dominant there is movement. If it is supported by *sattva* that movement will be clear, precise and in an intelligent direction; if it is supported by *tamas*, the movement will be unclear, misdirected or lacking conviction or purpose.

The second pair of interactions describe how the *guṇa* give birth to one another (*janana vṛtti*) and also contain the seed of the others within them (*mithuna vṛtti*). There is always a cycle of change. When a fruit is growing towards ripeness, we could say the predominant *guṇa* is *rajas*: it is moving towards wholeness. It has a sour taste and is sharp – both primary qualities of *rajas*. But within the predominant *rajas* are the seeds of the other two *guṇa* and as the fruit ripens, *rajas* gives birth to *sattva*. However, the dance of the *guṇa* does not stop here and before long, *sattva* itself gives birth to *tamas* as the ripe fruit begins to decay. Although this pattern of growth (*rajas*) leading to maturity (*sattva*) and then to decay (*tamas*) is common (and this applies to civilisations and yoga lineages as well as fruit!), it is not the only way the dance can play itself out. Sometimes *rajas* can lead directly to *tamas* with no intermediate step of *sattva*. *Janana* implies there is a constant change from one *guṇa* to another; *mithuna* implies that all three *guṇa* are always present at some level.

Finally, in SK 13, each *guṇa* is given two adjectives to describe its essential characteristic: *sattva* is said to be light (*laghu*) and luminous (*prakāśa*); *rajas* is stimulating (*upastambhaka*) and moving (*cala*); and *tamas* is heavy (*guru*) and obscuring, concealing or covering (*varaṇaka*).

	sattva	**rajas**	**tamas**
Nature (and effect on our minds) ***ātmaka***	Joy (*prīti*)	Pain (*aprīti*)	Despair (*viṣāda*)
Purpose ***artha***	Illumination (*prakāśa*)	Movement (*pravṛtti*)	Restraint (*niyama*)
Quality	Light (*laghu*) Luminosity (*prakāśa*)	Stimulation (*upastambhaka*) Movement (*cala*)	Heaviness (*guru*) Covering (*varaṇaka*)

Interaction of *guṇa*

Dominates (*abhibhavā vṛtti*)	Supports (*āśraya vṛtti*)
Gives birth to (*janana vṛtti*)	Contains within (*mithuna vṛtti*)

Polarities within *prakṛti*

As we have seen, at the highest level, Patañjali and Sāṃkhya propose a duality: the twin poles of *puruṣa* and *prakṛti*. One has form (*prakṛti*) and one does not (*puruṣa*); one is conscious (*puruṣa*) and one is not (*prakṛti*); one changes (*prakṛti*), the other does not (*puruṣa*). Some of these polarities are described in YS 2.5.[6]

If we focus solely on *prakṛti*, we will see how this is further divided into three. Three is very important – it is the minimum number to allow for a complex dance to arise. Each *guṇa* has a unique aspect which stands in contrast to the other two, and yet each is also similar to the others in different ways.

6. See Chapter 8.

- ***Rajas* and *tamas*** are sometimes described as *doṣa*[7] of the mind – they 'colour' our perceptions (*rajas* with passion, symbolised by red, and *tamas* with delusion, symbolised by black). Too much *rajas* and *tamas* is therefore undesirable because our minds are adversely affected. When *rajas* is excessive there is no stability, and when *tamas* is excessive there is no clarity. By way of contrast, *sattva* cannot be excessive, because it is pure and illuminating, and therefore cannot colour or stain.
- ***Rajas* and *sattva*** are by their very nature light and easily moved, whereas *tamas* is heavy. *Tamas* is able to provide boundaries and restraints; it gives structure, shape and form. Of course, this is essential and often helpful, but matter in the wrong place becomes 'dirt' that obscures or weighs us down, blocking our perception or our movement.
- ***Sattva* and *tamas*** are essentially inert; they do not move. It is only through the energy of *rajas* that *sattva* can grow or *tamas* can be moved and redirected. *Rajas* is the driving force which keeps the dance of *prakṛti* in motion. It can move us towards our goal, or it can move us away from it.

It is very important to understand that *guṇa* are not adjectives which describe aspects of *prakṛti*, or attributes of *prakṛti*: they **are** *prakṛti*. Very pleasingly, the word *prakṛti* is comprised of parts of the synonyms for the *guṇa*: *pra* (from *prakāśa*), *kṛ* (from *kriyā*) and *ti* (from *sthiti*) and the word itself thereby functions as a mnemonic to remind us that the *guṇa* are the fundamental ingredients of *prakṛti*.

The tools of transformation: Support, direction and space

Yoga has no concept of 'spiritual transformation' or 'spiritual growth' – because spirit (*puruṣa*) needs neither to transform nor to grow. In fact, it cannot – because it is unchanging. It is only *prakṛti* that we need to restructure and the project of

7. The word *doṣa* is commonly used in āyurveda to describe people's constitutions: it literally means 'that which colours or stains'. *Doṣa* is therefore something which is liable to 'go out of balance'; it is a fault.

yoga can therefore be seen simply as *guṇa* recalibration. The cultivation of *sattva* in the mind is a recurrent theme that runs throughout the Yoga Sūtra; indeed, the very highest stages of yoga are expressed by Patañjali in terms of the prevalence of *sattva* in the mind.

Support and *tamas*

For any project to be successful, there need to be solid foundations. Stability and 'givens' – things (people, ideas, structures) that can be relied upon – are vital. These are our **supports** whose function is to provide stability and structure. A support is something that we can rely upon to be unmoving when we lean on it; in order to 'take support' we must give something of ourselves to the support and trust that it will not collapse. A chair gives us support, the earth gives us support, a trusted friend can give us support. Here, we are using the concept of support as a synonym for the positive aspect of *tamas*: it is stable. Cultivating stability – finding and taking support – is the prerequisite to all growth. This works at all levels, from simple movements in āsana to the great journeys towards enlightenment. The first step is to 'prepare the ground' – and only then can we use the inertia and stability of *tamas* as a springboard.

Direction and *rajas*

Direction is a challenge. Sometimes it is clear, sometimes we are confused and paralysed by indecision: which path should we take? We have already seen (in Chapter 6) how in the *Bhagavad Gītā*, Arjuna was initially unable to act, caught between wanting to do the right thing and not wanting to engage at all. A direction requires a starting point and a goal. This may be a short-term goal or a long-term aspiration, but in order to get there, we must take intelligent steps in the right direction. In this sense, direction is part of *vinyāsa krama*. Because direction implies movement, we can also see it as an aspect of *rajas*. When direction is scattered, *rajas* is a *doṣa* (in the sense of being a fault); when our direction is clear and takes us towards our goal, we are using *rajas* appropriately because it is supported by *sattva*.

Space and *sattva*

In Chapter 4, we discussed the concept of *duḥkha*. *Duḥkha* is the starting point; it is the discomfort, irritation, restriction that causes us to seek change. Whether it is intense or just a background niggle, the presence of *duḥkha* is a reminder that our lives can change for the better. This does not necessarily mean a change in our external circumstances; sometimes (indeed often) it is a change of heart and mind. Whilst *duḥkha* is largely associated with restriction, its opposite, *sukha,* is experienced as openness. A clear **space** opens up. Although *sattva* is generally equated with light, we can also link it with a feeling of spaciousness. A lit candle dispels the darkness and thus gives us space to see.

Desikachar once described the process of meditation as "when *sattva* uses the stability of *tamas* to give direction to *rajas* to create more *sattva*".[8] We can see how this formulation can be directly superimposed on to Patañjali's very definition of the yoga project: *citta vṛtti nirodha*. The true nature of *citta* is *sattva,* but when *rajas* and *tamas* dominate, *citta* is out of balance. When *citta* is in its natural state, it is permeated with *sattva*, and it can use the stability of *tamas* (*nirodha*) to direct the movement of *rajas* (*vṛtti*). One could almost see it as a mathematical equation:

citta vṛtti nirodha (CVN) = sattva rajas tamas (SRT).

This formula can be expanded out to embrace the whole yoga project. Yoga's starting point is the feeling of *duḥkha*. Through yoga, we aim to open something within us to move towards *sukha,* a more spacious experience of the world. However, that movement needs to be carefully and skilfully crafted – experiencing 'states' is relatively easy, but turning states into traits takes time, commitment and practice. It requires a reorientation of our habitual tendencies. The

8. Personal communication.

path from *duḥkha* to *sukha* needs **support**: it needs to be held, cherished, preserved and protected. This requires boundaries. Once the boundaries are established there can be movement in a suitable **direction**; the boundaries are there to protect the practice and to lessen the tendencies towards dissipation (too much *rajas*) or inertia (too much *tamas*). When we see clearly, we see what we need to restrain and how we can move. The more space (*sattva*) there is, the more beneficial the workings of support (*tamas*) and direction (*rajas*), resulting in yet more **space**.

> *We use the support (nirodha) of tamas to give direction (vṛtti) to rajas, to open more space for sattva (citta)*

This simple formula can apply to āsana, prāṇāyāma, meditation, chanting, devotional practices, food – even our relationships with our teachers or indeed the Tradition itself. It is at the very heart of our understanding of the journey of yoga.

Two directions: *Bhoga and apavarga*

Is the cultivation of *sattva* and the consequent feeling of spaciousness enough? It is certainly the prerequisite; flooding our being with *sattva* is the aim of the practices described by Patañjali in his famous eight limbs of yoga (*aṣṭāṅga*). But the danger of stopping here, according to both yoga and Sāṃkhya, is, as we have seen, that we get stuck in the realms of the Gods, and forget our journey. We become too comfortable. Moreover, the *guṇa* dance will continue; just because we are in a space of *sattva* today, doesn't mean that *tamas* and *rajas* won't dominate tomorrow as we are caught up again in the whirligig of *guṇa* fluctuation.

YS 2.18 finishes with two possible directions which our experiences can take us towards: *bhoga* or *apavarga*. *Bhoga* means 'enjoyment' – not necessarily in the sense of pleasure, but meaning that we enjoy the fruits of our karma: we get what we get. *Bhoga* is experience to be experienced;

it is food to be digested. It is only through ingesting that we grow. We need experiences in order to realise our place in the world and to help us be our best possible selves. But equally, experience has the potential to corrupt: too much, too soon, or inappropriate experiences which remain unprocessed can act like poison, leaving us with 'mental indigestion' that results in bitterness, fear or resentment. It is a fine line to walk, but the practice of yoga and the cultivation of *sattva* can be a huge help in maintaining our stability and navigating the potentially difficult experiences that we have to face throughout our lives. So, the first step is to deal most elegantly with our experiences, to creatively and skilfully engage with *bhoga*.

But Patañjali offers another step, which is not just about dealing with *bhoga* but about transcending it altogether: *apavarga*, meaning 'liberation' or 'emancipation'. Any experience, any aspect of nature, can be used as a means of transcendence. When we have experienced something sufficiently to know that we don't need to repeat it, we have understood that particular lesson, digested and outgrown it, then we have achieved (to some degree), liberation. This step necessitates *vairāgya*, the ability to remain free within certain situations; to minimise unhelpful and automatic reactions (usually involving desire or aversion). Even *sattva* has a pull, a gravitational weight to it, and for Patañjali the ultimate goal is to be completely free within the dance of *prakṛti*, irrespective of whether *sattva, rajas* or *tamas* dominates. Our centre has moved sufficiently from the fortress of our constructed self to allow a far more transparent mode of Being where we are no longer impelled to act out our habits and compulsions.

The word order here is very important; *bhoga* comes before *apavarga*.[9] We need experience to digest, only then can we transcend. We cannot say that we are 'above something' if we have never tried it or experienced it.

9. In the same way, *abhyāsa* comes before *vairāgya*, *sthira* comes before *sukha* and *tapas* and *svādhyāya* come before *īśvara praṇidhāna*. This formulation runs throughout the sūtras: work, prepare, act, and then release.

Experience requires us to engage, process and then to move on, and it is our responses that determine whether we are further embroiled or moving towards liberation. Desikachar puts it simply: "The World exists to set us free."[10] Responding with *vairāgya* is the movement from *bhoga* to *apavarga*.

Sādhana: Dynamic and static āsana

One of the most important supports that we have when we come to practise āsana is the depth of the tradition. We can refer back to our teachers, and also to the wealth of literature that has enriched our understandings and our practice. We know that Patañjali has defined yoga as *citta vṛtti nirodha* (YS 1.2, see Chapter 1), but Desikachar has given us a very simple and structured *vinyāsa* which takes us towards this goal. "Without āsana practice, prāṇāyāma cannot be mastered. Without *prāṇa nirodha,* mind will not become stable."[11] Thus, we need āsana to contain the body (*kāya nirodha*), then prāṇāyāma to contain the breath (*prāṇa nirodha*), and finally we contain the mind (*citta vṛtti nirodha*). He ordered the progression in this way because we start with the grossest, most tangible and therefore the easiest to manipulate (the body), and finish with the most subtle (the mind).

What does it mean to 'contain the body'? To us, this means holding the body (relatively) still for a reasonable length of time in order to embody the qualities of *sthira* and *sukha* in a static posture.[12] This requires strength, stability and flexibility. To obtain these qualities, it is very useful to work with the breath, and to work with dynamic postures first as a preparation for static āsana. Looking at ancient texts like the *Haṭha Yoga Pradīpikā*, there is scant information on *vinyāsa krama*. For example, this is how it describes the lotus posture (*padmāsana,* fig 7.1):

10. This is the title of Chapter 12 of Desikachar's book, *The Heart of Yoga* (op. cit).

11. This is from Desikachar's commentary on Krishnamacharya's version of the Yoga Rahasya, *Krishnamacharya Yoga Mandiram,* 1998.

12. See Chapter 9 for more detailed discussion on *sthira* and *sukha*.

"Place the right foot on the left thigh and the left (foot) on the right thigh, cross the hands behind the back and firmly take the toes (the right toe with the right hand and the left toe with the left). Place the chin on the breast and look at the tip of the nose. This is called padmāsana; it destroys all diseases..." HYP 1.46. [13]

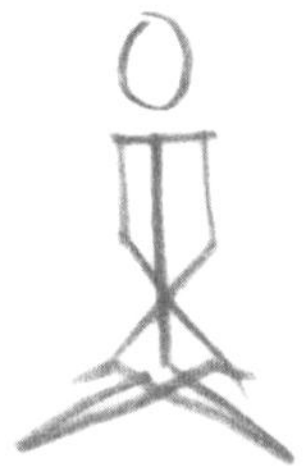

fig 7.1

And this is how the symmetrical seated forward bend (*paścimatānāsana,* fig 7.2) is described:

"Stretch out both legs on the ground without bending them, and having thus taken hold of the toes of the feet with the hands, place the forehead upon the knees and rest thus. This is paścimatānāsana" HYP 1.28.

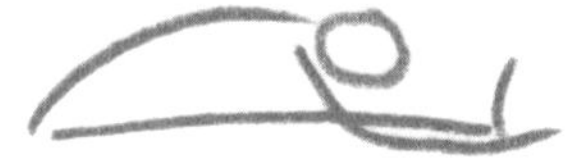

fig 7.2

Apart from the minimal detail on the route in and out, the texts are often very scant on how long one should stay in postures, or the order of postures and so on. In the ancient Sanskrit texts, there is little emphasis on dynamic āsana; postures are described as positions to stay in (often for a very long time) in order to cultivate meditative absorption. However, this emphasis on static āsana highlights the dangers of taking ancient texts too literally, especially if you don't have a teacher to help deconstruct them and make their teachings digestible and practical. For most people, straining to stay in something like the lotus posture in the

13. This is actually a description of what we now call *baddha padmāsana* – the 'bound lotus'.

hope of gaining immortality is simply delusional and will not engender *sthira* and *sukha*: it will simply damage the knees!

Krishnamacharya was very precise in his teaching about dynamic āsana. In the modern Western world, the term 'dynamic' is sometimes equated with 'strong' or 'intense'; but this is not the meaning we intend here. We understand the term dynamic to simply mean 'moving' – practising a posture dynamically means moving in and out of the form. What is the function of dynamic āsana, and why did Krishnamacharya stress its importance?

Dynamic postures involve large movements of the body. Moving completely in and out of the posture is a full-range movement (fig 7.3); we can also have mid-range movements (partial movements in and out of the posture, fig 7.4) and even micro-movements (subtle movements made while maintaining the posture, fig 7.5). These movements help to warm and train the body (and attention) to move slowly and carefully into and out of the pose. In other words, working dynamically prepares the body to stay in the pose. Mid-range and micro-movements can follow full-range movements of the body as we refine and intensify our practice:

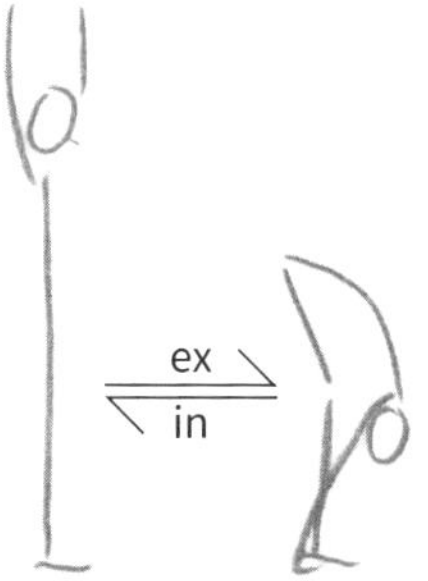

fig 7.3

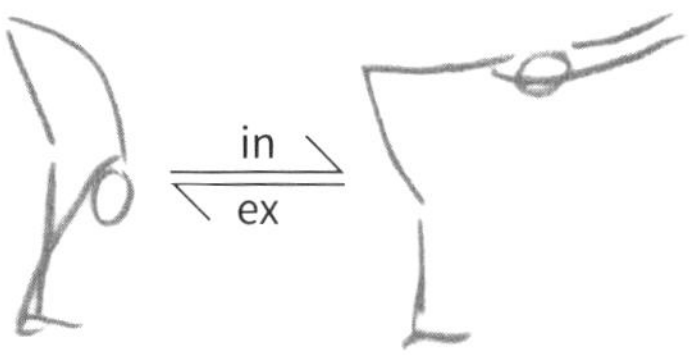

fig 7.4

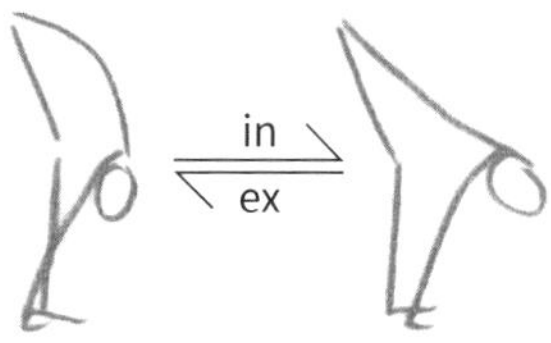

fig 7.5

There is another good reason to use dynamic posture work as preparation for static. If you are travelling at 50mph in a car and then suddenly slam on the brakes, the contents of the car will continue to move although the car has stopped. Similarly, sitting still after you've been rushing around with a busy mind can sometimes actually amplify your perception of the busy mind. If instead you change down through the gears as you move from 50mph to a standstill, the contents will slow at the same rate as the vehicle and by the time the vehicle comes to rest, so too does the driver. Dynamic work not only prepares the body physically, but also gives the attention a support; instead of the mind being dissipated it can focus on the movement. By giving the mind something tangible to hold on to, the mind is being harnessed and directed. So, at a psychological level too, dynamic work is also a good preparation for static work.

Finally, it is worth comparing our ability to breathe in a static āsana with our breath in a dynamic one. Most people will find their breath far more compromised when staying in a posture than when moving in and out. This is because if we work intelligently with the breath, synchronising it with appropriate movements of our limbs and torso, the breath will actually support the movements of the body and the movements will support the breath.[14] For example, a movement into a forward bend will compress the abdomen and push the diaphragm upwards into the thoracic cavity facilitating an exhalation. Similarly a movement into backward bend lifts the ribcage and expands the chest, facilitating an inhalation. It is the movement into and out of the postures that facilitates the breath; once you're in the posture retaining the same slow deep breath is often more challenging. Once again, we have a compelling reason to start working dynamically prior to static āsana.

14. See Chapter 9 for more on breath in āsana.

Chapter 8

अविद्यास्मितारागद्वेषाभिनिवेशाः
क्लेशाः ।
अविद्याक्षेत्रमुत्तरेषां
प्रसुप्ततनुविच्छिन्नोदाराणाम् ।

Kleśa: *Avidyā*'s Different Forms

YS 2.3 avidyā-asmitā-rāga-dveṣa-abhiniveśaḥ kleśaḥ

Misunderstanding (avidyā), confused sense of self (asmitā), habitual desire (rāga), habitual aversion (dveṣa), and profound fear (abhiniveśa) are the afflictions (kleśa)

YS 2.4 avidyā kṣetram uttareṣāṃ prasupta-tanu-vicchinna-udārāṇām

The ground (kṣetra) in which all afflictions grow, is misunderstanding (avidyā). These afflictions can be dormant (prasupta), weak (tanu), truncated (vicchinna), or fully mature and reproducing (udāra)

One of the ways to understand a new concept is through the use of metaphors, similes or analogies. We describe something new with reference to what we already know. Although no metaphor is perfect, by imposing previous understandings onto a new concept, we are able to see it (or some aspect of it) more clearly and our comprehension slowly grows. A common contemporary metaphor for the mind is a computer – people talk about 'reprogramming' their minds, or 'downloading' new ideas. Patañjali uses images from nature in tune with a more rural and agricultural culture.

In YS 2.3, Patañjali simply lists the *kleśa*. Often translated as the 'afflictions', they run throughout life and are felt by all to various extents at different times. They are part of what it means to be alive. There is a very significant order to the list, and we can consider how these afflictions relate to each other and how they may manifest in the body. Arising out of misunderstanding (*avidyā*) comes a confused sense of self (*asmitā*) to which we cling. This is a misidentification with something ephemeral (like our current thoughts or feelings). By clinging to this feeling, we make an idol out of shadows; there is nothing permanent there. This feeling of self is perpetuated by habitual likes and dislikes (*rāga* and *dveṣa* respectively). Like an engine, *rāga* and *dveṣa* power the creation and continuity of identity and 'feeling of me'. And running through all of these afflictions is a thread holding it all together: fear (*abhiniveśa*).

In the next sūtra, YS 2.4, Patañjali goes on to describe the grounds for them all as a field (*kṣetra*). This is the field of misunderstanding (*avidyā*). Out of this field, other afflictions can grow and they, too, will have different stages in their lifecycle. Patañjali outlines four potential states of *kleśa*: dormant (*prasupta*), weak (*tanu*), truncated (*vicchinna*) or fully mature (*udāra*).

When dormant and unseen (*prasupta*), they are like seeds in the ground. We think there is no problem, and yet – given the right conditions – a desire or an aversion can suddenly sprout and begin to show itself. As a seedling, the affliction is stretched thinly, it is weak (*tanu*). Here there is a 'thin fuzz' of new growth, as the plants begin to develop. They are still easily managed, but their very presence shows that the soil contained seeds. The '*kleśa* plant' can continue to develop in the soil but before it reaches full maturation it can be cut down (*vicchinna*), or eclipsed. This is usually because another affliction overrides it: the desire for one thing (an ice cream) may be obscured because of a fear of something else (a spider in the way). By the time the plant becomes fully mature (*udāra*), we are no longer in control – it dominates us. Not only that, but having come into flower it can now spread its seeds to further perpetuate the cycle of *karma*. This fully mature stage of *kleśa* is extremely dangerous to our equilibrium; our decisions and actions are clouded by imbalances, and our minds inevitably become a breeding ground for yet more imbalance and affliction by propelling us into further actions based in *kleśa*.

Understanding the *kleśa* in more detail

We have already seen how the heart of the yoga project concerns the mind rather than the body, and the source of our suffering is our misunderstanding. It is extremely important to grasp that *avidyā* is *misunderstanding*, and not simply a lack of understanding or ignorance. *Avidyā* is far more profound than that; it is unconscious. We can be consciously ignorant of something – I *know* that I don't speak Spanish. This is not *avidyā*, because in a state of *avidyā*, we do not realise what we don't know. This is why *avidyā* is so difficult to detect – it is utterly unconscious and we are unaware of it. It is, in effect, our blind spot, and according to Patañjali, this blind spot is at the heart of our very existence (until we wake up). In this way, *avidyā*, and the resulting *kleśa*, permeate our lives.

Defining *avidyā*: Specific confusions

YS 2.5 anitya-aśuci-duḥkha-anātmasu nitya-śuci-sukha-ātma-khyātiḥ avidyā

Confusing the impermanent, the impure, the limited and non-essential with the permanent, the pure, the spacious and the essential is avidyā

There are many ways in which we can be confused or wrong, many potential arenas for our misunderstanding. But Patañjali defines *avidyā* in very specific terms by presenting four pairs of opposites – and in each we back the wrong horse. These are:

I	II
anitya (impermanent)	*nitya* (permanent)
aśuci (impure)	*śuci* (pure)
duḥkha (limited, restricted)	*sukha* (unconfined space)
anātma (non-essential)	*ātma* (essence)

Avidyā is a way of seeing. It is the specific misunderstanding that gives birth to the four other *kleśa* and it is defined as the confusion of the second column with the first. Thus, we project qualities from column II onto column I, thereby denying the reality of column I.

We give permanence (*nitya*) to the impermanent (*anitya*); we think the impure (*aśuci*) is pure (*śuci*); we believe the limited (*duḥkha*) is unlimited (*sukha*); and finally, we superimpose essence (*ātma*) onto what is simply not there (*anātma*). It is interesting that the word *khyāti* (embedded in *ātmakhyāti*) means both to 'perceive' and to 'declare'. In a state of *avidyā*, we perceive qualities of *ātma* or *puruṣa* in our bodies and minds and declare this to be the case by acting as though it were true. This is misperception. The reason that this is *avidyā* is because our minds and bodies are subject to change and thus subject to *guṇa*. Because they change, decay and die, they are in the realm of *prakṛti*, whereas what we are projecting onto our bodies and minds are the qualities of *puruṣa*.

Each of the pairs is significant. The first pairing reminds us that there is nothing permanent in our experience. Not only does every cell of the body continuously change, but so do our thoughts, our feelings of who we are, our moods, our very perception of the world. Sometimes I feel like a good person, sometimes I feel bad! Confusing the impermanent for the permanent, we could sum up this first pair thus: *we refuse to accept change.*

Is there an implicit morality in the second pairing? Does Patañjali imply that we must 'purify' our impure bodies through some kind of ascetic denial? We can consider our bodies (and minds) 'impure' in so far as they need maintaining: they need cleaning and looking after. If they were inherently pure, they would need no maintenance. Moreover, we tend to cloak our fallibilities with 'purity'. All too often, we deny or repress unwholesome feelings or motivations and thereby fail to acknowledge an aspect of our humanity. We are not perfect![1] We could sum up this

1. And interestingly and paradoxically, at the level of *puruṣa*, we also *are* perfect already!

second pair, of confusing the impure for the pure, thus: *we refuse to accept our shadow.*

We have translated *duḥkha* as 'limited, or restricted' (space), whilst *sukha* is 'unconfined space'. These are more commonly understood as 'pain' and 'joy' respectively, but *duḥkha* is really about the pain, frustration or suffering that arises when we feel constricted or limited. *Sukha* is its opposite; it is the feeling of open, free and easy space. Interestingly, however, the feeling of too much space can be just as disorientating as too little. Too much choice, for example, can also be overwhelming.[2] As incarnated beings, we necessarily have to exist within limits – we are to some extent confined by our physical limitations and these limitations increase as we grow older. What is important, however, is that form and structure (and therefore limits) need not be perceived as prison walls. The structure of a haiku or a sonnet define the poem's limits; once those limits have been understood and accepted, they can be used creatively and harnessed to become supports. However, if we rail against limits, misunderstand boundaries or think the world *should* be otherwise, we simply bang our heads on walls in unrealistic utopianism. We could sum up this third pair, of confusing *duḥkha* and *sukha*, thus: *we refuse to accept our limits.*

The final pair suggest that we give a solidity and form to something that is simply not there. Ascribing essence (*ātma*) to that which is not there (*anātma*), gives rise to defensiveness, hostility, and a feeling of being 'up against the world'. In this state, we see our skin as the end of our territory, and everything inside that skin (including the thoughts and feelings that are produced by our current state of being) needs defending against the ravages of what lies outside. Ultimately, it's a losing battle. We deny the possibility that there is anything beyond our superficial understandings and cling to the idea that the reality we exist in is the only one possible. We could sum up this last pair, of confusing *ātma* and *anātma*, thus: *we refuse to accept depth* – and thus we are happy to be anaesthetised by the superficial.

2. Supermarkets are notoriously well known as places for people to suffer panic attacks. Sometimes the sheer variety of possibilities can be too much and we become paralysed by confusion and fear.

The four aspects of *avidyā* can appear somewhat abstract and impenetrable, but by seeing them as four refusals[3] we can see how they play out in our lives:

- *we refuse to accept change*
- *we refuse to accept our shadow*
- *we refuse to accept our limits*
- *we refuse to accept depth.*

These refusals appear unconsciously in our attitudes and motivations and thereby drive our actions without our awareness. Although shining a light on their presence may begin to lessen their impact, simply knowing about them is not necessarily enough: they are unconscious forces at the heart of how we think and act.

Patañjali asserts that until we fully wake up, *kleśa* will colour our lives, and behind all *kleśa* is *avidyā*. We could go as far as to say that actually there is only one *kleśa* – *avidyā* – and these four are simply its various manifestations. Yoga's concern, therefore, is the clarification of *avidyā*.

Asmitā: A false identification with the energy of life

YS 2.6 dṛg-darśana-śaktyoḥ ekātmatā iva asmitā

When the energy of the Seer becomes confused with the process of seeing, a false identity arises

Without a sense of self, life would not only be intolerable, it would be unliveable. We need to have an identity in order to interact with others, to give us perspective on our experiences and to coordinate the many functions of our body-mind. The term Patañjali uses for 'sense of self' is *asmitā*, but it's important to appreciate that this has two forms: *asmitā rūpa* and *asmitā kleśa*, and only the latter is pathological. *Asmitā rūpa*[4] simply means 'the feeling of one's Self'. However, when we (mis)identify that feeling

3. Insights arising from Peter Hersnack, personal communication.

4. For further discussion around *asmitā rūpa*, see YS 1.17.

and become glued to concepts of who we are, this becomes a *kleśa*. So, in YS 2.6, Patañjali deepens his discussion of *avidyā* by clarifying how it manifests as *asmitā kleśa*. *Asmitā kleśa* is fundamentally a confusion. It is seeing two things as one: *iva* means 'as if' and *ekātmatā* means 'one (*eka*) essence (*ātma*)'. Here, the power of the Seer (*dṛg śakti*) is confused with the faculty for perception (*darśana śakti*) – that is to say, with our senses and our minds. A 'pseudo Self' is created from the very real feeling of being alive. By projecting identity onto thoughts and perceptions, the illusion of form and continuity crystallises around mental fluctuations. Our work, our relationships, our likes and dislikes become who we think we are. *Asmitā kleśa* is a very serious state: it is a heavy burden which may manifest as a furrowed brow, hypersensitivity, and a feeling of discomfort, anxiety, arrogance or defensiveness in our own body.

Rāga and *dveṣa*: Replaying our past desires and aversions

YS 2.7 sukha-anuśayī rāgaḥ

Rāga is the desire to repeat previously pleasurable experiences.

YS 2.8 duḥkha-anuśayī dveṣaḥ

Dveṣa is the desire to avoid previously painful experiences

Just as not all feelings of self are pathological, so not all desires or aversions are problematic. The desire for water when we are thirsty, or the repulsion towards things which are dangerous to us, is natural and healthy. Patañjali talks about a specific type of desire and a specific form of aversion – these are called *rāga* and *dveṣa* respectively.

In some senses, *rāga* and *dveṣa* are opposites of one another. Common to both of them is the term *anuśayī*, which means 'flowing on from' and implies a tendency towards repeating experiences. *Rāga* is defined as the desire to repeat pleasurable experiences, whilst *dveṣa* is the attempt to avoid previously painful experiences. What makes them *kleśa* is that they are not based in present time, but in past conditioning. Even if we want something new, the desire is a replay of a past habit: we might want a new piece of technology, but the pattern of desire is the same old, same old. *Rāga* and *dveṣa* 'replay' desires: they both arise from *asmitā kleśa* and also perpetuate it.

Rāga can be seen as a form of addiction – many drug addicts have talked about how their addiction stems from the desire to repeat their very first experience of a drug. Unfortunately, this is a doomed venture: we cannot repeat it and feel the same way because we (and everything else) have changed. This is a replay that endeavours to take the experience out of the present, like trying to taste fruit we dreamed we ate. Although it may feel that we are giving ourselves what we desire (and thereby supporting ourselves), it is actually illusory. We trick ourselves into chasing after the unreachable.

In the same way, *dveṣa* is also out of the present time. *Dveṣa* is a re-run of a previous unhappy experience and it shuts us down from the present moment because we are heavily conditioned by our prejudices against whatever stimulated our aversion in the first place. We may wish to avoid something – but in doing so we become trapped. While running away from our fears may reduce our anxiety momentarily, eventually we simply paint ourselves into a corner and have nowhere to hide. *Dveṣa* is the *illusion* of really being free.

It is interesting to reflect on the nature of play. Play is an 'as if' experience – it is both serious and also light. When children play, they are completely absorbed in the experience: it is their present. At its most profound, play takes us 'out of time' and in this sense, is unlike 'replay' which is very much in time. Thus sportsmen and women are so utterly engrossed in the present moment that thoughts of yesterday or tomorrow are irrelevant (indeed, such thoughts would interrupt the flow). We are not suggesting those in a 'flow state of play' have permanently undermined *asmitā*, but we can say that at that moment, it is greatly reduced. Perhaps this is one of the reasons that sport, and indeed any experience of heightened presence (enthralled dancing, listening to music, singing) can feel so good: it takes us out of our habitual confined sense of self and opens us to a far more transcendent and spaciousness sense of Being. These experiences are 'liberating'. One antidote therefore, to the seriousness of *asmitā kleśa*, and the replay of *rāga* and *dveṣa* is simply to play: be present, light of heart, and engaged.

Abhiniveśa: Clinging to life

YS 2.9 svarasa-vāhī viduṣo'pi samārūḍhaḥ abhiniveśaḥ

Abhiniveśa is a clinging to the 'feeling of oneself' and is experienced even by the wise

There is an instinctive reaction towards preservation of life against death. Our autonomic nervous systems quickly fire up when we are in danger – we gasp if our breathing is compromised, we flinch from something which burns, we fight to stay alive when there is a threat to life. As long as we are alive, this fear of death will operate at some level simply because it is hard-wired in us. The traditional commentators of the Yoga Sūtra see *abhiniveśa* as exactly this fear of death. The word *vāhī* means 'carrying' or 'bearing'; *svarasa* is 'one's own juice'. The first word of the sūtra, *svarasavāhī,* therefore means 'holding (onto) one's vital fluid'.[5] *Abhiniveśa* is defined as the 'clinging to (this tendency)' and it affects everyone equally (*samārūḍhaḥ*) – even the highest sage, a *viduṣaḥ.*

5. Because we are made up mostly of water, this means we cling to our bodies, our incarnated selves.

Relationship between *kleśa*

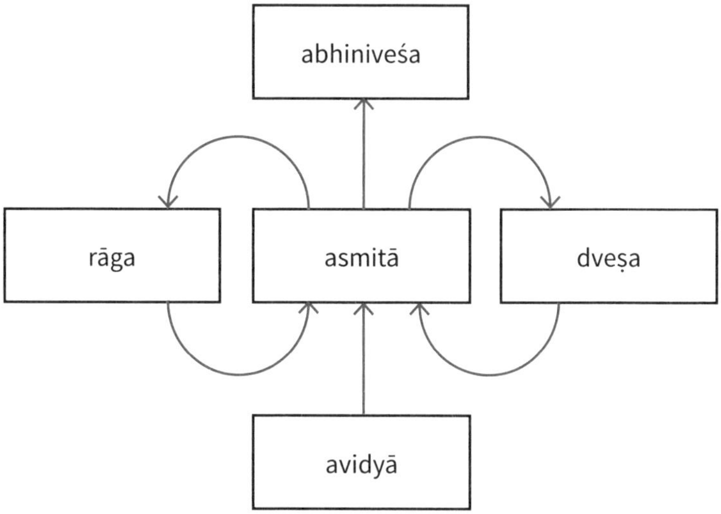

Some say that because *abhiniveśa* is experienced by all, it means that *kleśa* are also fundamental to the embodied experience. *Avidyā* is certainly seen as a common experience for everyone who has yet to awaken to *vidyā*, but let us not confuse *abhiniveśa* with a generic autonomic reaction to danger or a general fear of death. Instead it can be understood as a very specific fear arising out of protecting a false identity. It is how we feel when we are so wedded to our own identity – our views, ideas and habits – that any change or threat provokes a profound fear and resistance. *Abhiniveśa* is the fear of letting go, of being challenged or destabilised. As long as there is *avidyā*, there will be *asmitā*, powered by *rāga* and *dveṣa*, and if there is *asmitā*, there will be *abhiniveśa*. *Asmitā* is like 'constructing (and inhabiting) our castle'; *abhiniveśa* arises when we feel the threat of eviction![6]

As we have seen, the *kleśa* will not be dominant (*udāra*) all the time; it is quite possible, indeed probable, for the *kleśa* to be weak (*tanu*) or even dormant (*prasupta*) until circumstances conspire to push the *kleśa* into a more noticeable manifestation. However, importantly, we should

6. Peter Hersnack described it as "the fear of being uninstalled".

acknowledge that these different levels of *kleśa* are natural – and sometimes *kleśa* will be overwhelming. This is not an indication of us failing or being 'bad'; it is simply part of a natural cycle. And remember: things change and what is overwhelming now will once again retreat to a *tanu* or *prasupta* state in due course.

Uprooting the *kleśa*

YS 2.10 te pratiprasava-heyāḥ sūkṣmāḥ

These five kleśa are subtle and are overcome by a return to their original state

Yoga is sometimes described as 'swimming upstream'. The very first limb of *kriyā* yoga is *tapas*[7] – that is, purifying actions that challenge us. *Tapas* requires us to go against our habitual patterns and to swim upstream. In using the term *pratiprasava* (the second word of the sūtra), Patañjali alludes to this concept since *prati* means 'against' and *prasava* means 'the flow'. We can therefore understand the term as a sort of backtracking, of retracing one's footsteps back to the source. From a traditional perspective, *pratiprasava* is the process of moving our attention from the most external and grossest parts of our being (our physical form, our senses) though progressively more subtle aspects (the various parts of our mind) until we have flooded the whole system with a clarity born of *sattva*.

'Returning to the source' is not historical. In other words, it is not about going back in time. *Pratiprasava* is not concerned with intra-psychic archaeology – digging around for clues in our earliest memories. A slightly unusual way of understanding this 'returning to the source' is becoming present to this very moment, becoming aware of the *right now*. As we have seen, we can understand this presence as an antidote to *kleśa,* which are fuelled by the endless replay of *rāga* and *dveṣa*. Becoming alive to the present moment is the opposite of 'spinning out' into fears, desires, aversions

7. If we see *kriyā yoga* as a preliminary to *aṣṭāṅga yoga*, then we can also say that the beginning of *aṣṭāṅga* is *tapas* too. It is the basis for the yoga project. For a detailed discussion of *kriyā yoga* see Chapter 13.

and fortifying one's sense of entitlement. It is the simple and profound realisation that we are here and now, and that *kleśa* are built upon *avidyā* – an elsewhere which, by disguising itself as reality, usurps it.

Understanding and managing the effects of *kleśa*

YS 2.1 dhyāna-heyāḥ tadvṛttayaḥ

Through meditation (dhyāna), the causes of afflictive mental activity (vṛtti) are overcome (heya)

What is the route to this elusive present moment? How do we swim upstream? Here, Patañjali equates the *kleśa* with their mental symptoms – the (*citta*) *vṛtti* – and states that the way to both understand and manage their effects is *dhyāna* (meditation). In *dhyāna,* we begin to settle the mind's activity by focusing on a single object (*dhāraṇā*), and as that process stabilises, the mind's tendency towards 'spinning the wheel of *kleśa*' is reduced. The gravitational pull of the *kleśa* weakens as we reorient ourselves. Ultimately as we remain in the practice, *dhyāna* evolves into *samādhi* and profound insights arise as well as a loss of sense of self. The present moment shines and replaces the usual thoughts, distractions and feeling of 'self-consciousness'.[8]

Saṃyoga and *kleśa*

YS 2.17 draṣṭṛ-dṛśyayoḥ saṃyoga heya-hetuḥ

Confusing the Seer and that which is seen is the cause of the suffering that is to be avoided

We have seen (in Chapter 4) how we can understand *saṃyoga* as embodied *avidyā*. The state of *saṃyoga,* as described by Patañjali in this sūtra, is thus a consequence of *avidyā*. This state can include how we hold ourselves, how we move, how we interact and even how we think.

8. This process is explored in more detail in Chapter 13.

Fundamental to yoga is an understanding of space and difference; yoga is concerned with the creation of a space which enables a good relationship. *Saṃyoga* is its opposite: space is compromised and boundaries become blurred.

In any space that joins two principles – the space between bones in the body, between married couples, between children and parents, between body and mind – unwanted material can accumulate. In āyurveda, undigested material which is not expelled is called *āma*. As *āma* accumulates, it begins to overflow and circulates in the system, lodging itself wherever it finds a free space. Once it is has become embedded, it begins to compromise that space so that instead of a free relationship, it creates an unhealthy singularity. Although *āma* is generally considered a physical substance, we can think of a psychological and emotional equivalent. Undigested thoughts, feelings and experiences can also accumulate and lodge themselves in our system. Eventually, this unprocessed material can severely compromise the health of a relationship; the free space between the two principles becomes a confused space where the autonomy of each principle is lost and where identities become blurred. Pointing to the problem, each side blames the other.

In a healthy joint, two bones slide freely in relationship to one another, allowing the space between them to be uncomplicated. Where there is pathology, this space becomes compromised, manifesting as pain and limited movement. Toxins (unwanted material) restrict the space, creating discomfort or pain. In effect, the two bones are no longer able to work interdependently, but rather only work as one – when one moves the other is affected.

In the same way as bones or other parts of our bodies can become 'stuck' together, so we can become 'glued' to outdated ideas or perceptions that block us from seeing the reality of the present moment. We become fixed in our own preconceptions. And from an interpersonal perspective, a couple can become so used to each other that they no longer see each other for who they are. Accumulated and habitual ways of interacting block clear and fresh perception, and the relationship loses its vitality and becomes stale.

This state of confusion is called *saṃyoga* – literally 'complete joining in a confused way'. Just as *avidyā* can look like *vidyā* (because it is a *wrong* understanding rather than *no* understanding) so *saṃyoga* can look very much like yoga (because it is *wrong* relationship rather than *no* relationship). It is 'yoga in disguise', an attempt at maintaining a relationship which is failing because of the accumulated detritus of the past. What should not have been joined has become as one; two principals have become inseparable and confused. In the state of *saṃyoga,* space is compromised resulting in a feeling of restriction, loss of vitality and an inability to move or interact freely. This is *duḥkha*.

Sādhana: Moving from *saṃyoga* to *viveka* in body and breath

The key principle of yoga which helps us overcome *saṃyoga* is *viveka*: the ability to see things from both sides, to discern. *Viveka* is a fundamental requirement for yoga, and our initial steps on the path help us to cultivate this discriminating awareness. When we are ignorant about a particular subject, it is very difficult to make any judgements about that subject (although of course, many people do!). Someone who knows nothing about jazz may be unable to distinguish the sound of Charlie Parker from that of John Coltrane. It is only through experience and practice (in this case, of listening) that we begin to develop an understanding of how, where and what to distinguish. As this understanding deepens, we are able to make finer and finer judgements, and so cultivate *viveka*.

Saṃyoga in the body

When someone first comes to a yoga class, they are likely to have poor body awareness unless they have had training through another discipline like T'ai Chi, dance or Alexander Technique. Perhaps because our culture is so mental (in both senses of the word), many people are disconnected from their bodies, and function like disembodied heads on trolleys. Bodies are something, as the educator Ken Robinson graphically put it, "to take you from one meeting to the next."[9] It is no surprise, therefore, that making subtle adjustments to the spine, or being aware of the movement of the shoulder blades, or noticing the relationship between the knees and the hips is a total mystery for the novice yoga practitioner. To begin with, sensations need to be fairly gross for them to register at all. This common experience for beginners is a form of *saṃyoga* because everything seems to move together, but not in a harmonious or conscious way. The beginner's body often moves as a single block.

The innovative body-mind therapist Moshe Feldenkrais often described unconscious movements that accompany conscious ones as 'parasitic': they 'feed off' a host movement. As we refine our practice, we learn to inhibit these unconscious and unnecessary movements, which can confuse transmission of lines of force, making the body work harder because it is pulled in more than one direction. For example, if we bring our knees over the chest when we are lying down, we might find our chin lifting, thereby compressing the back of our necks, and our sacrum coming off the ground resulting in a rounding of the lower back.

If the body is working against itself, the support for the movement is obscured and the direction becomes confused. By removing unnecessary twitches, tensions, or movements we are able to create a cleaner direction that enables clear transmission from a stable base.

This process is more akin to sculpture (the removal of unnecessary material to reveal an essence), than painting (in which something is created by being 'built up'). The

9. A particularly striking image from Ken Robinson's TED talk 'Do Schools Kill Creativity?' (2006).

saṃyoga of movement, therefore, is the unconscious and inefficient use of the body where true support for the movement is eclipsed, resulting in excess and unnecessary effort. The ability to simplify a movement, such that we create a stable base and then move in a clear direction, is to apply *viveka* in āsana.

Saṃyoga in three polarities

We can poetically describe three polarities which, while not being exactly equivalent, do nonetheless have a certain thematic consistency. The first of these is simply the two fundamental principles of yoga and Sāṃkhya: *puruṣa* and *prakṛti* (fig 8.1):

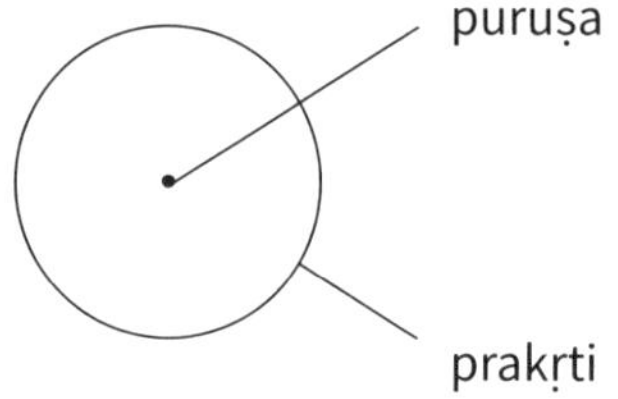

fig 8.1

We are taking a bit of a liberty by representing *puruṣa* as a dot in a circle because, actually, it is out of time and out of space, and certainly not confined 'within' *prakṛti*. However, with imagination we can see how this diagram represents one aspect of the polarity between the observer (*puruṣa*) and that which is observed (*prakṛti*). At its most global and profound, *saṃyoga* is exactly the confusion between these two polarities: this is the fundamental *avidyā*. It lies at the very heart of the philosophy of yoga and Sāṃkhya. As you practise, ask yourself: can you create the time and space to notice how the body moves and to observe, without becoming enmeshed?

In the texts of Haṭha Yoga, another pair is introduced which reflects something of this initial polarity. This pair defines the vertical axis in the body: at the top is the head, symbolised by the moon (*candra*) and at the bottom is the pelvis, symbolised by the root (*mūla*) (fig 8.2).

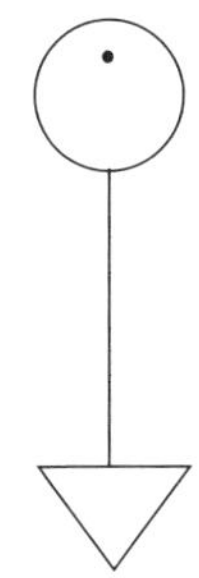

fig 8.2

Candra is a synonym for the highest, most subtle part of the mind, called *buddhi*, whose function is to discriminate. In the yoga tradition, it is seen as that which reflects the light of *puruṣa* (just as the moon reflects the light of the sun). It is not exactly the same as *puruṣa,* but it can be thought of as a sign – how the light and awareness of *puruṣa* manifest in the body. At the other end is the pelvis which contains the densest bone of our body, the sacrum. This end of the vertical axis is *mūla,* which literally means 'root'. It contains our 'tail' (the coccyx) which symbolises our roots in humanity and even the animal kingdom – and is thus something of a reflection of *prakṛti*. The ascent through the vertical axis is thus a symbolic journey from the grossest aspects of the material world through to the most rarefied and subtle realms of spirit. Because they are two ends of the spine, how one end moves affects the other and consequently there is tremendous potential for unconscious or 'parasitic' movement in the head or pelvis as one or the other move. In our practice, can we become sensitive to the relationship between the movement of the head and the movement of the pelvis?

The vertical axis is two-dimensional, and it cannot exist alone in space. It needs a container to take it into three dimensions. We can further elaborate this essential polarity

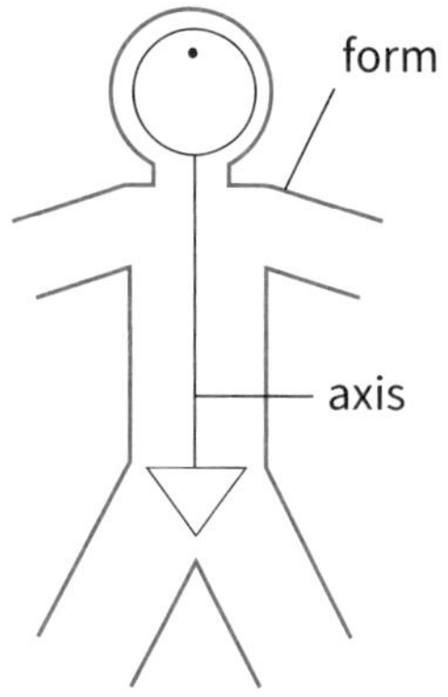

fig 8.3

by contrasting the vertical axis and the form within which it abides (fig 8.3).

It is wrong to equate the axis with *puruṣa,* but in construing an imaginary line around which our form dances, we can say that something of *puruṣa* is reflected in the axis. Similarly, although the form is not pure *prakṛti,* it *is* what we can directly observe (the way we are in the world, how we hold ourselves and how we manifest), so it can be seen as a reflection of *prakṛti.* It is a useful exercise to practice āsana with full concentration on the axis, or full concentration on the form, and indeed sometimes with full concentration on their relationship.

Try this simple sequence (fig 8.4), first focusing on the axis, then the form, and finally on the relationship between the two:

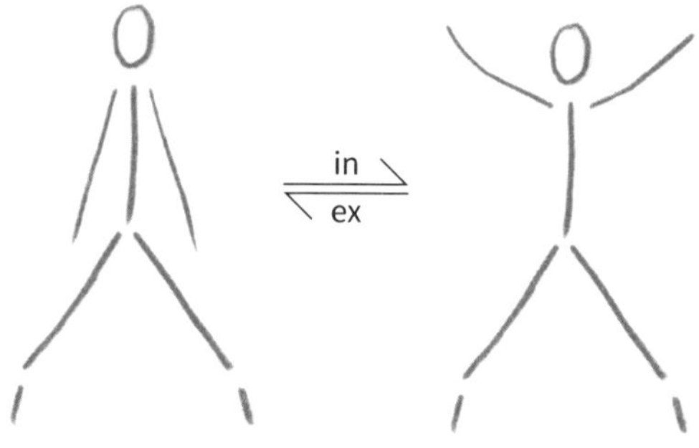

fig 8.4

At its most sophisticated, when yoga is really working, the axis is both supported by and a support for, the form; just as *puruṣa* is both supported by and a support for *prakṛti*.

Saṃyoga of the body and breath

Novices are often confused about the coordination of breath and movement in āsana, but with practice, it does not take long to intuit whether a movement should be performed on an inhalation or an exhalation. As we have seen, the basic rule of thumb is that any movement in which the abdomen is compressed (primarily forward bends and twists) should be performed as we exhale, and actions which cause the sternum to lift or the ribcage to expand (primarily backward bends) should be performed as we inhale. As practitioners become increasingly experienced, the breath and body begin to settle into a very comfortable relationship and get to know each other pretty well. There's a feeling that because we are raising the arms, we need to be inhaling; because we are folding forward, we need to exhale. This sort of bodily intuition is necessary and in many ways desirable, but like all relationships, it comes with a potential problem: familiarity allows us to switch off. Sometimes (particularly with experienced practitioners) the body and breath can look like they are working together: both are smooth, even and long, but despite appearances, they are not really in relationship. Instead, both breath and movement have an automatic quality and the relationship has become dull, habitual and unconscious. Neither surprises one another.

The challenge therefore is to keep the relationship fresh and to avoid this 'pseudo-relationship' of *saṃyoga*. One way of challenging this is to become very sensitive to the habitual movements of the body as we inhale and as we exhale. Notice the shoulders, the spine, the head and the hands. Do they move with the breath? Does that movement support the breath, or is it simply an unconscious result of the breath? Sometimes it is worth keeping an area fixed and stable despite a habitual tendency, as if the body were saying to the breath: "You do your thing, but I'm going in this direction!" This sort of separation between breath and movement is a form of *viveka*, and can re-invigorate their relationship with freshness and dynamism.

Chapter 9

स्थिरसुखमासनम् ।

Practising Āsana

YS 2.46 sthira-sukham āsanam

With the correct stability in a posture, spaciousness arises

This succinct statement contains three words: *sthira, sukha* and *āsana*. The first word, *sthira,* relates to English words like 'stay', 'stability' and 'still'. It implies a certain effort required to remain. The second word, *sukha*, is a beautiful word which can be further divided into its two component syllables: *su* and *kha*. When *su* is used as a prefix in Sanskrit, it indicates something pleasant and comfortable. The word *kha* refers to space (often specifically the space in the heart – and therefore an emotional experience of space). So *sukha* literally means a pleasing space, a space in which we are easy and comfortable. (We have already discussed its opposite, *duḥkha*, sometimes translated as suffering or pain, in Chapter 4).

There are many ways to translate this sūtra into English. Here are a few:

- *The posture (should be) steady and comfortable*
  – Georg Feuerstein[1]
- *Āsana must have the dual qualities of alertness and relaxation*
  – TKV Desikachar[2]

- *The postures of meditation should embody steadiness and ease*
  – Chip Hartranft[3]
- *The posture is firm and comfortable*
  – Frans Moors[4]

It is important that *sthira* comes first; after all, *sthira* is the effort we put into cultivating stability in the posture. If the effort is correct, and appropriate, the fruit will be *sukha*. Too much effort or wrong kind of effort (for example, gritting your teeth or clenching your jaw) will simply lead to *duḥkha*. Likewise, without a certain amount of *sthira* a posture is not really fully formed: flopping into a posture in a casual and mindless way – even if it looks good from the outside – is not āsana.

1. Feuerstein, Georg: *The Yoga Sūtra of Patañjali*, Inner Traditions International, 1979.

2. Desikachar, TKV: *Patañjali's Yogasūtras: An Introduction*, Affiliated East-West Press Ltd, 1987.

3. Hatranft, Chip: *The Yoga Sūtra of Patañjali*, Shambhala Classics, 2003.

4. Moors, Frans: *Liberating Isolation*, Media Garuda, 2012.

The importance of āsana in modern yoga practice

Of all the practices offered by Patañjali, it is undoubtedly āsana that has captured the modern imagination. Indeed, many now equate āsana with yoga; the American yoga teacher Gary Kraftsow reflected that "yoga has been reduced to āsana and āsana has been reduced to stretching".[5] While purists may despair, there is something to be said for āsana as a primary vehicle or methodology of yoga, especially in an increasingly sedentary world where we can easily become displaced from the physical realities of our bodies. At its best, āsana can help us re-integrate and to become more fully embodied.

The dancer Martha Graham once said that "dance is the song of the body".[6] If that is the case, then āsana can be its poetry. We can see this in the very names of postures. Sometimes they take the form of mythological people or animals (*vīrabhadra,* the mythical warrior; *ananta,* the mythical serpent; *naṭarāja,* the Lord of the Dance; *cakravāka,* a mythical bird). At other times the name refers to an animal (*adho mukha śvānāsana,* downward-facing dog posture; *bhujaṅgāsana,* cobra posture; *śalabhāsana,* locust posture; *siṃhāsana,* lion posture; *kūrmāsana,* turtle posture). Sometimes a natural form is invoked (*tāḍāsana,* the mountain or *padmāsana,* lotus posture). Each of these invites us to express something of the name of the posture in the ways we exercise its form; we give the shape of our body an extra dimension by embodying metaphor.

Peter Hersnack took this idea even further. He taught that when we have become fully embodied, the āsana functions 'as a sign' – that is, something which points to something *beyond* itself, which we can't necessarily perceive directly. Peter described how āsana "is work that enables something deep within us to express itself".[7] This beautiful idea evokes something of *puruṣa*; the *form* of the posture is an indication of the truth and reality (*sat*) of the awareness

5. In an interview with Anna Dubrovsky, *Yoga + Joyful Living*, Spring 2009.

6. Thanks to Ranju's twin brother Sanjoy Roy for this quote, from the 'Planet Dance' series of animated shorts (Planet Dance, 2015). www.youtube.com/watch?v=AUZ9a06fOKg.

7. Personal communication, Launde Abbey 2006.

(*cit*), and the peaceful joy (*ānanda*) that is its essence. It is very difficult to capture this in a photograph; but each individual person has the possibility of expressing something of this living essence every time they practice āsana.

Defining āsana

How do we know what is and what isn't a yoga posture? Is it enough to adopt a particular pose, to place our limbs and trunk in a certain way? When we look at ancient texts on yoga, it comes as quite a surprise to find that āsana, far from being what yoga is all about, has a relatively minor role in traditional practice. Instead, āsana is seen as a means to an end. There are two important functions of various āsana discussed in ancient texts such as the *Haṭha Yoga Pradīpikā*: firstly, as postures for meditation, and secondly, for manipulating the energies (rather than the anatomy) of the body. The purpose of this purification and energetic manipulation is primarily to promote spiritual experiences, but certain health benefits also arise

In most ancient Sanskrit texts on Haṭha Yoga (which were composed in the last six hundred years or so) we find that the first function – that of adopting a suitable position for meditative practices – is by far the most common. In the fifteenth-century text, *Haṭha Yoga Pradīpikā*, fifteen postures are described in detail, nine of which relate to cross-legged seated postures in some form. However, many of these are also seen as optimum postures for manipulating energies of the body – particularly along the vertical axis, and thus could be seen as promoting spiritual experiences as well as health.

There are some rather extravagant claims made about the health benefits of some of the poses, and these claims should be taken with a pinch of salt. Thus, for example, *paścimatānāsana* (the seated forward bend) is said to "stimulate the gastric fire, make the loins lean and destroy all the diseases of men" (HYP 1.29).[8] The author of the *Haṭha Yoga Pradīpikā*, Svātmārāma, even went as far as to say that

8. *The Haṭhayogapradīpikā of Svātmārāma*, The Adyar Library and Research Centre, Madras 1972

mastery of certain techniques will confer immortality on the diligent practitioner after a certain amount of regular practice: "The knower of yoga, who being steady, has the tongue turned upwards and drinks the soma juice doubtless conquers death in fifteen days" (HYP 3.44). However, as Krishnamacharya is said to have wryly commented, where is Svātmārāma now? You may not achieve immortality, but what is for sure is that an intelligent approach to the practice of āsana will have numerous health benefits. Āsana practice can lead to extraordinary levels of physical prowess and may also function as a wonderful therapeutic tool.

Since the nineteenth century, the number of āsana has dramatically increased, and this is undoubtedly linked to the growth of yoga's popularity in the West. Teachers and schools invented and 'discovered' new forms, new ways of coming into postures and new sequences combining postures. If a posture only has an English name and doesn't have a Sanskrit one (e.g. dolphin posture), it is likely to be a relatively recent invention.[9]

There is undoubtedly a certain one-upmanship that can be seen in the contemporary yoga world when people talk of practising 'classical āsana'. It gives us the impression that a particular form has preordained qualities, and the execution of that form confers a certain level of spirituality and authenticity to the practitioner. In *Yoga Body*, Mark Singleton assesses the impact of the photograph on the understanding and practice of āsana.[10] Singleton argues that the still photograph moves us away from the private sphere and into the public: "Yoga – or a rather particular, modern variant of *haṭha* yoga – began to be charted and documented through photography with something like the 'objective stance of the pathologist' (Budd, 1997:59)". Postures became objectified and the photograph could be used to illustrate their 'ideal form' (according to whichever authority one adhered to). This represents a movement from the embodied to the iconic.

In BKS Iyengar's hugely influential *Light on Yoga*,[11] the forms of the āsana become reified into the 'classical' or

9. It's worth noting that Sanskrit names are not evidence of antiquity in āsana. There are many postures, for example, *trikonāsana* and *adho mukha śvānāsana*, which seem to be comparatively modern postures despite their Sanskrit names. The Sanskrit names have been 'retro-fitted' to modern forms.

10. Singleton: *Yoga Body* op. cit. see Chapter 8 pp. 163–174.

11. Iyengar, BKS, *Light on Yoga*, George Allen & Unwin, 1966.

iconic postures to which we must aspire. Photos can be useful up to a point, but with them comes the danger that we struggle to emulate an external form rather than understand the essential *function* of a posture and then intelligently adapt it to suit our own capacities – physical, psychological and emotional. In other words, we must be clear to distinguish **function from form** such that the form can be appropriately and intelligently modified to respect function.

So, it is difficult to say what is or what is not a yoga posture: looking at photos in a book or magazine is not the answer. However, we will endeavour to first describe certain conditions that need to be met for a bodily posture to be a yoga āsana, and then the various ways in which they can be met. In YS 2.47, Patañjali gives us perhaps the most open, broad, and yet incisive, definition of āsana: *sthira-sukham āsanam.*

The dynamic relationship between *sthira* and *sukha*

Although we have already begun to explore how *sthira* is the starting point and *sukha* is the fruit, we can develop our understanding considerably by seeing how these two qualities differ depending on the āsana, and also how they interact with each other during the different phases of the breath.

Certain postures are intrinsically *sukha* in their quality. Where is the effort to remain in a posture like *śavāsana* (the corpse pose, fig 9.1)?

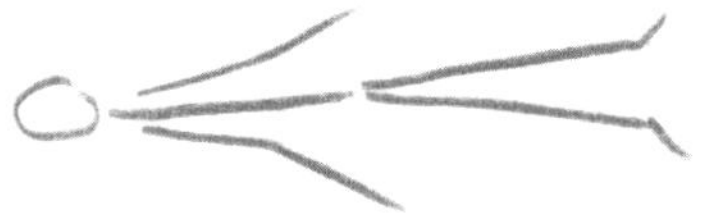

fig 9.1

Because the body is completely relaxed, there is no *sthira* required in the musculature. However, importantly, there must be *sthira* of the attention, and movement should be contained. For *śavāsana* to fulfil the conditions of āsana, we must remain present and alert and not just drift off to sleep. Thus, the qualities of *sthira* and *sukha* can apply as much to attitude as to physical effort. Let us contrast *śavāsana* to a much more physically demanding posture like *dhanurāsana* (the bow, fig 9.2).

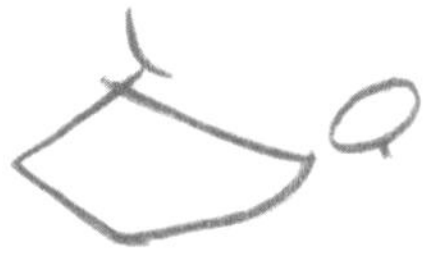

fig 9.2

Here, tremendous muscular effort is required – the challenge is to approach the posture (both physically and psychologically), sufficiently lightly to let the quality of *sukha* manifest. Only then does the posture open gently like a flower, so that although it is physically strong, it is also pleasing and comfortable. Just as the strings of a musical instrument require the right amount of tension, so too, each posture requires the right amount of *sthira*. Too tight is wrong, too loose is wrong; just right produces the perfect note: *sukha*.

However, it is also important not to think of *sthira* and *sukha* as static ingredients in the composition of āsana (Peter Hersnack joked that āsana is not about "30 grams of *sthira* and 30 grams of *sukha*"!)[12]. They do not simply 'balance each other', leading to a sort of mutual cancelling out. This is a way of 'domesticating' the postures; instead they should dance together, give birth to one another, be in constant dynamic play with each moment. This interaction between *sthira* and *sukha* is mediated by the breath. As we inhale, part of the body remains firm and stable (**support**), another part moves (**direction**), opening out into **space**. Usually on the inhalation the firm part (*sthira*) is the abdomen, the

12. Personal communication.

pelvis and perhaps the legs. This stability allows the spine to lengthen and the space between the head and the pelvis to open (*sukha*). This reverses as we exhale: often there is an effort to remain open as we exhale lest there is a collapse of space in the trunk. This effort to keep the form open during the exhalation is *sthira*. Usually this *sthira* of the exhalation is in the upper part of the body (head and chest and particularly in the sternum), and it allows the abdomen and hips the freedom and space to move.

The essential method

YS 2.47 prayatna-śaithilya ananta-samāpattibhyām

Through skilful effort we can loosen the knots of being and let ourselves be supported by breath

This is a fascinating sūtra with layers of meaning and interpretation, but essentially it gives us the methodology for achieving *sthirasukham āsanam*. It is divided into two parts, *prayatna-śaithilya* and *ananta-samāpatti*. Both are essential. The grammatical case-ending (*bhyām*) implies instrumentality and duality; in other words, **both** *prayatna-śaithilya* and *ananta-samāpatti* are the **means** by which we achieve *sthira* and *sukha*.

Prayatna is a special, committed (*pra*) type of effort (*yatna*): it is an effort in which we invest something of ourselves; we are intensely engaged. *Śaithilya* is the state of being loosened and relaxed. The first part of the sūtra suggests that we make a special effort to come into a state of relaxation, to loosen the knots of our Being (physical, mental, emotional).[13] This is effort that transforms itself into ease.

The second part, *ananta-samāpatti*, is also divided into two parts. *Ananta* means 'without end', infinite. It can also be used as another metaphor for the breath:[14] rather than seeing us as breathing, we see the whole universe as

13. This interpretation of the term *ananta* is another way in which Krishnamacharya taught this sūtra; and undoubtedly it is idiosyncratic. Other traditions understand this sūtra slightly differently – we have chosen this interpretation as it is at the heart of this way of working.

14. According to the Nyāya school (a sister philosophy to yoga and *Sāṃkhya*), there are three types of prayatna (effort): *pravṛtti, nivṛtti* and *jivanaprayatna*. Here the latter, *jivanaprayatna*, is implied – this refers to the effort of breathing. Thus, *prayatna-śaithilya* can be understood as 'the effort to make the breath smooth and even (*śaithilya*)'. This is how the long-time student of Krishnamacharya, Srivatsa Ramaswami, taught this sūtra.

breathing and us as 'being breathed'. Breath goes far beyond our individual confines: it is infinite. In this way, we can see *ananta* as another name for *prāṇa*, the vital energy of the universe, the breath of all living creatures. *Pat* means 'to fall'; adding the prefix *ā* implies that we fall towards something (*āpatti*). Peter Hersnack suggested that we fall 'inwards'. Finally, *sam* means 'together' or 'completely'. Thus, *samāpatti* implies we fall completely, we release into, we move closer towards... what? We fall inwards towards the essence of the breath: *ananta, prāṇa*.

In one of the most famous and popular stories of Indian mythology, the gods (*devas*) and the demons (*asuras*) needed a rope to churn the Milky Oceans to extract the Elixir of Immortality (*amṛta*). As a churning rod, they used Mount Meru, the great mountain which stands at the middle of the world (and is sometimes likened to our spine, forming the central axis). They lifted and inverted it, so that its tip was deep in the ocean. But what could be used as a

'The breath is a mediator which can help to bring opposites to work together towards a common purpose.'

churning rope that was strong enough, flexible enough and long enough to coil around Mount Meru and be held by those opposite forces, the *devas* and the *asuras*? They used Vāsuki, the great Serpent, who is also sometimes equated with the King of the Serpent deities, Ananta. Vāsuki/Ananta is that which enables opposites to work together towards a common goal. Likewise, in the practice of both āsana and prāṇāyāma, the breath is a mediator which can help to bring opposites to work together towards a common purpose (yoga).[15] The breath can bring into relationship the left and the right, the top and the bottom, the front and the back, the axis and the form. *Ananta* enables a joint project.[16]

Applying this understanding to the sūtra, we can see how *anantasamāpatti* can be construed as taking support

15. In the practice of prāṇāyāma, Mount Meru can be seen as the spine, the nostrils represent the *devas* and the *asuras*, and the breath itself, moving from one nostril to the other, is Ananta/ Vasuki.

16. It's also worth noting that *ananta* as breath (or more accurately, *prāṇa*) not only enables a joint project, but is also the product of a joint project. *Prāṇa* is understood to be the product of the interaction between *puruṣa* and *prakṛti*. It is *puruṣa's* proximity to *prakṛti* which generates *prāṇa* – when *puruṣa* leaves, the body dies and *prāṇa* dissipates.

on the breath/*prāṇa*, which in turn supports us. This leads to a profound question regarding the complete sūtra when applied to āsana: what effort can I make (*prayatna*) to enable the conditions (*śaithilya*) for me to take support (*samāpatti*) on that which carries me (*ananta/prāṇa*)? And for those interested in this tradition, when considering this question in relationship to āsana, the answer is clear and simple: to work skilfully with the breath. The work of āsana thereby becomes an exploration and a meditation on *prāṇa* and its movement within the body.

The fruit of āsana

YS 2.48 tato dvandva-anabhighātāḥ

Then we are not overwhelmed by the pairs of opposites

We have seen how, in keeping with Indian tradition, Patañjali divides the world of phenomena into three strands: *tamas*, *rajas* and *sattva*. In āyurveda, the three *guṇa* are fleshed out into twenty qualities called the *gurvāḍi guṇa*.[17] These twenty qualities are actually ten pairs of opposites: heavy/light; hot/cold; unctuous/dry; gross/subtle; static/dynamic; dense/flowing; slow/fast; soft/hard; smooth/rough; and finally, gelatinous/clear. With these ten pairs, āyurveda is able to describe many of the qualities of *prakṛti* – from the cold, hard, sharp qualities of icicles to the soft warmth of feelings of love. Thus, even thoughts, feelings and memories can be described by the *gurvādi guṇa* in the same way as physical objects.[18]

Patañjali goes on to describe the fruit of mastering āsana as the ability not to be overwhelmed by the pairs of opposites. At a physical level, āsana gives us a certain resilience, an ability to withstand the wider fluctuations in external conditions. We are able to remain more tolerant towards extremes of both cold and heat. In certain ascetic traditions, yogis of old would sit unmoving in icy streams, or surrounded by fire in the midday sun. This is an intense form

17. *Gurvādi* means '*guru* (heavy) and the rest' – in other words, it implies a list with *guru* at the beginning. A teacher is sometimes called 'guru' because they have gravitas; they are literally 'heavy' with knowledge.

18. There are actually other qualities described in āyurveda, some relating directly to the mind and feelings. Thus intellect, memory, desire, hatred and happiness are all described as *guṇa* in *Caṛaka Saṃhitā* Vol 1 v49.

of *tapas*: the ability to withstand external demands and remain focused on our goals, to stand firm. Even now there are extraordinary stories of yogis who meditate in the freezing cold of the mountains, or remain motionless for days on end.[19]

Without going to these extremes, we can see how the practice of āsana can help build resilience and stability and thereby render us less susceptible to the vagaries of external conditions. Āsana can also help us with moods, emotions and thoughts. They can help to centre us, so that we are less unsettled by success or failure, by happiness or grief. By reducing our tendency to fall out of balance, āsana can optimise our stability and enhance not only our physical, but also our mental health.

Sādhana: Breath and āsana

Breath and spinal position

One of the hallmarks of this approach to yoga is the focus on the breath. It is precise, logical, considered and refined. For Desikachar, it was of primary importance and without its sensitive application, something profound is missing from āsana practice. As we have said, breath brings potentially disparate elements into relationship; it yokes mind (attention) and body (form). In this sense, breath *is* yoga. Desikachar was very insistent that when practising āsana, body and breath should be synchronised. Certain movements are to be performed as we inhale, others as we exhale. To synchronise the breath is to make the breath *at least* as long as the movement; ideally we practise in a way that makes the breath 'frame' the movement so it starts slightly before the movement begins and finishes just after the body has come to stillness. Furthermore, the breath should remain long, slow and smooth with an even quality throughout. An uneven, ragged breath is a sign that

19. In *Roots of Yoga*, for example, James Mallinson and Mark Singleton describe a contemporary yogi in India who once a year remains utterly motionless for nine days continuously.

we are over-exerting ourselves; the breath thus functions as a mirror.

In YS 2.50, Patañjali introduces us to the components of the breath.[20] The order in which he introduces them is significant: first, the exhalation, *bāhya vṛtti* (moving outwards); then the inhalation, *abhyantara vṛtti* (moving inwards) and finally *stambha vṛtti* (holding the breath, either in or out). We start with the exhalation because it 'clears out'; it 'wipes the board clean'. The correct exhalation facilitates the subsequent inhalation by providing stability, particularly in the abdomen. The inhalation has then got something to 'work against'; the firmness of the abdomen created at the end of the exhalation is like a springboard from which the inhalation can find direction. In this way, the exhalation provides support for the inhalation, and thereby allows a space to open up.

The breath is developed by bodily movements. Forward bends in particular help to lengthen and refine the exhalation. In a forward bend, the hips close, the abdomen compresses and the diaphragm is pushed upwards into the chest cavity. Like the plunger of a syringe, this forces the air up and out, helping us to exhale. Not only does the body help the breath, but the breath helps the body. As we exhale, the body becomes less rigid – think of inflating and then deflating a balloon. Because of this, we are able to soften and relax into forward bends as we exhale. If we take a forward bend on an inhalation, the result is horrible – like driving with the foot on the accelerator and the brake at the same time! Because forward bends support the exhalation so well, they are often the first group of postures we work with. They help us to develop both the stability and the flexibility to deepen our āsana practice and broaden our range of postures.

As with forward bends, the exhalation also facilitates spinal rotation, so we move into twists as we breathe out. In full twists, the abdomen (often) becomes compressed and a degree of flexibility is required. The body is 'wrung out' like a dishcloth and this requires us to exhale. Inhaling into

20. See Chapter 10.

a twist is like inhaling into a forward bend: uncomfortable and counter-productive.

Backward bends, where the front of the body opens and lifts, are usually performed as we inhale. The inhalation lifts the sternum, broadens and lifts the ribs and helps us to open into the posture. When the movement of the spine is against gravity (as in *bhujaṅgāsana* or *śalabhāsana*), the inhalation can give the body support: the body can 'fly on the thermals' (this also works as we come out of a standing forward bend). Sometimes however, inhaling into a backward bend can cause compression and a feeling of tightness in the back (we are, after all, becoming more rigid as we inhale). In such cases, and particularly when there is back discomfort, weakness or pathology, it can work very well to exhale into backward bends (fig 9.3), and then stay there for the subsequent inhalation helping to further open and lengthen the posture.

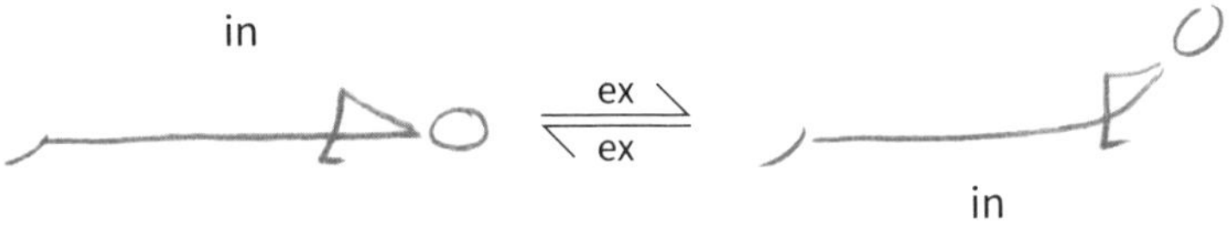

fig 9.3

Prāṇa and *apāna vāyu*

The ancients subdivided the energy *prāṇa* into five subcategories called the *pañca prāṇa vāyu* ('the five wind energies'). These subcategories of energy perform different functions within our system. They are responsible for the healthy functioning of our bodies and indeed it is said that the difference between a live person and a corpse is the presence of *prāṇa*. Of these five, two are particularly linked to our breath: *prāṇa vāyu* (rather confusingly this has the same name as the more generic *prāṇa*) and *apāna vāyu*. They are not exactly the same as the inhalation and the exhalation, but the inhale particularly influences *prāṇa vāyu*, and similarly the exhale particularly influences *apāna vāyu*.

Prāṇa vayu's home (*prāṇasthāna* – the place of *prāṇa*) is located in the chest. As we open and lift from the chest when we breathe in, it is as if the breath originates from the heart, expanding in all directions from its home. Similarly, *apāna vayu's* home is in the lower abdomen below the navel, where the body becomes firm at the end of an exhalation. Their functions are also different: *prāṇa vayu's* role is to connect, to link, to open new spaces and directions. *Prāṇa vāyu* is linked to the future; it is an 'adventurer'. *Apāna vāyu*, on the other hand, cleans up. Whereas *prāṇa vāyu* links and is future-orientated, *apāna* separates and is more past-orientated in the sense that it removes rubbish; it 'clears away dirt'. *Apāna vāyu* is intimately linked to our past because the more that 'stuff' accumulates, the harder *apāna vāyu* has to work – and sometimes it just becomes overwhelmed. Because *prāṇa vāyu* and *apāna vāyu* 'have the same bank card', as it were, they draw from the same energetic account.[21] If *apāna vāyu* is overspending, *prāṇa vāyu* has fewer resources. When we are overrun with accumulated waste from the past which we haven't got rid of, we have less energy for new ventures and experiences: we are just too tired. This is another reason why we work on the exhale – and thus *apāna vāyu* – first.

Two types of inhale, two types of exhale

While postures that open the chest and favour the inhalation can be classified as '*prāṇa*' postures (also known as *bṛṃhaṇa kriyā*), and postures favouring the exhalation can be classified as '*apāna*' postures (also known as *laṅghana kriyā*), not all breathing works with the same energetic intensity and efficiency. It is useful to distinguish between two types of inhalation and two types of exhalation.

An inhalation that *fills* is very different from an inhalation that *opens*: it occupies space rather than opening it. The more we fill as we breathe in, the tighter we become and at the end of the breath we feel completely blocked: there is nowhere left to go. This is a crude inhalation that

21. This formulation is another of Peter Hersnack's many insights.

creates rigidity as it grasps and holds on. However, we can also inhale in a much more subtle way in which we 'open from inside' rather than 'filling from outside', and this gives a completely different feel to the practice. It is as if we could go on breathing in forever: the movement feels like a continuous yielding and opening from within. Interestingly, when a baby is born, the lungs and trachea are 'flat packs' – they are vacuum-sealed. Our first breath is thus not a 'taking in' but an 'opening up'. We open to the world to receive it rather than simply filling up from outside. This opening gives *prāṇa vāyu* the space to do its work.[22]

We can also distinguish between an exhalation that 'collapses' and one that 'separates'. Peter Hersnack joked that exhalation isn't simply "a retention of the breath with a slow puncture." This just leads to deflation, and *apāna vāyu* is unable to function efficiently, because there is no space for it to circulate. In order for *apāna vāyu* to be able to function there needs to be a differentiation between the exhalation and the form of the posture; it is as if we hold the form open as we breath out and, like a receding tide, the exhalation withdraws back to its home. If we vacuum clean a rug that is lying on a wooden floor, we have to hold the rug still in order for the cleaner to work (that is, to separate the dirt from the rug). If we don't, then the rug will simply move with the vacuum cleaner and there will be no separation. This is the equivalent of an exhalation that collapses: nothing happens on an energetic level. In both of these examples (an inhalation which opens and an exhalation which remains open), *there is a palpable distinction between body and breath.* They interact with each other in a profound way, but they also remain free. In the contrasting types of breath, where the inhalation fills and the exhalation collapses, body and breath are 'glued' to each other, and are thereby imprisoned.

22. It is interesting to reflect on the emphasis given in Haṭha Yoga to the free circulation of *prāṇa* and the removal of blockages that impede it. Free circulation requires space that is not full of 'other stuff'.

Ujjāyī in āsana

The basic methodology of breathing in āsana within this tradition is *ujjāyī*, sometimes called 'throat control breathing'. Desikachar described *ujjāyī* as "that which clears the throat and masters the chest".[23] Its literal meaning is 'giving mastery over the upward (movement)' and at a bodily level, *ujjāyī* acts as an expectorant, helping to dry excessive dampness from the trachea and thereby 'master' the chest.

In *ujjāyī*, we create a restriction in the throat and there is a gentle hissing sound – it feels as if we are breathing directly in and out through the throat. This gentle friction, created by the turbulence as the flow of air passes through the restriction, can be used as a support for the movement, for the breath and for the attention. As a support for the movement, *ujjāyī* gives 'body to the breath': it makes the breath more substantial and helps the body float on its presence. As a support for the breath, *ujjāyī* helps to lengthen the breath, to make it more subtle and refined. Very importantly, we make a distinction between *ujjāyī* and the breath: *ujjāyī* is a tool which refines and controls the breath, but they are not the same. At its most subtle, we could even say that *ujjāyī* is a *sign* of the breath, an indication of the quality of the breath. Finally, as a support for the mind, *ujjāyī* gives the attention a tangible place to settle upon; it creates a gravitational pull that helps to keep the mind from scattering.

As *ujjāyī* is used throughout āsana practice, it becomes the default breath. But – and it's a big but – it has the potential to be abused. If *ujjāyī* becomes too habitual, we can easily switch off to it and it becomes an 'alibi': "Yes, I was present! I was doing *ujjāyī*!" While it can really help new practitioners to focus and refine their āsana practice, there is a potential danger for any experienced practitioner that it simply becomes a habit. For this reason, it may be helpful to use images and suggestions to keep our relationship with *ujjāyī* fresh. *Ujjāyī* can be seen as 'a place of contact', as

23. TKV Desikachar, *Religiousness in Yoga: Lectures on Theory and Practice*, eds. John Ross Skelton and Louise Carter (Lanham, Maryland: University Press of America 1980), p. 119.

'touching the whole body and not just the throat'; or indeed 'a caress not a control'. It is easy to make the breath too rigid. Instead, we should let the breath play a little, to watch the interaction between breath and body and let that interaction be surprising sometimes, so that one moves in one way and the other in another. This helps maintain a freshness and joy with each breath we take in our āsana practice. Our ability to habituate, appropriate and abuse our relationship with what begins as being a genuine support is everywhere – yoga easily becomes *saṃyoga*!

Finally, although *ujjāyī* is the default breath in our practice (particularly in āsana and prāṇāyāma), it should not be practised throughout the session nor as the default breath in our daily lives. When we are resting in between postures, or in *śavāsana*, for example, we should be able to let the breath be natural and unforced. We should also appreciate that in meditation, the breath is usually free and it is important, therefore, to be able to let it go as appropriate.

Chapter 10

तस्मिन् सति श्वासप्रश्वासयोर्गतिविच्छेदः
प्राणायामः ।

Practising Prāṇāyāma

YS 2.49 tasmin-sati śvāsa-praśvāsayoḥ-gati-vicchedaḥ prāṇāyāmaḥ

Established in this (āsana), prāṇāyāma is regulating the flow of the inhalation and the exhalation

As with the sūtras on āsana, Patañjali takes the topic of prāṇāyāma and breaks it down into a definition (YS 2.49), a methodology (YS 2.50), and its fruit (YS 2.51, 2.52 and 2.53). However, there are at least three ways of understanding this sūtra in which Patañjali defines the basic parameters of prāṇāyāma practice. The first words, *tasmin* and *sati* mean that 'something has been established'. Because this sūtra follows on immediately from those discussing āsana, it is clear that Patañjali is referring to a posture that has the qualities of *sthira* and *sukha*. To practice prāṇāyāma properly, we need to feel comfortable in our seated posture so that we can remain undistracted. Prāṇāyāma cannot be effective if we are concerned with the pain in our knee, or with a slouching spine and a collapsing chest. Nor can it arise if our minds are too distracted – there needs to be stability and freedom in both the body and the mind.

The next words, *śvāsa* and *praśvāsa,* can be understood in two different ways. At the most basic level, *śvāsa* simply means 'breathing in' and *praśvāsa* means 'breathing out'.

However, the terms are only used on one other occasion in the whole text (YS 1.31), and this is in the context of Patañjali's description of the symptoms of experiencing obstacles. In YS 1.31, *śvāsa* and *praśvāsa* are not simply inhalation and exhalation, but the type of unconscious breathing which arises when we are experiencing suffering; in other words, Patañjali is describing an uneven, ragged and disturbed breath.

Finally, the last term, *gativiccheda,* is made up of two words. *Viccheda* means 'cutting' or 'stopping'; whilst *gati* implies a movement or a flow. When we combine this with the previous term (*śvāsapraśvāsa,* with its two meanings), a number of possible interpretations arise. First of all, if we understand the term *śvāsapraśvāsa* to refer not simply to the inhalation and the exhalation, but to a habituated, ragged, and disturbed breath (YS 1.31), then prāṇāyāma can be seen as stopping the flow (*gativiccheda*) of unconscious, poor breathing patterns (*śvāsapraśvāsa*) and instead cultivating a conscious and regulated way of breathing.

However, if we consider *śvāsa* and *praśvāsa* simply to mean 'inhale' and 'exhale', we can also say that prāṇāyāma is 'regulating the flow of the breath' – it is how we 'cut' (*gativiccheda*) the different parts of the breath, how we divide the inhalation and the exhalation. This leads us to an understanding of prāṇāyāma as an exploration of breathing ratios – the length of time an inhalation takes compared to that of the exhalation. This is, of course, a fruitful area of study and practice, about which more later.

Finally, we may consider *gativiccheda* to literally mean 'stopping' or 'arresting' the inhale and the exhale. This implies the cultivation of the pauses between inhaling and exhaling, or between exhaling and inhaling. Prāṇāyāma is thus the retention of the in-breath (called *antaḥ kumbhaka,* or 'AK') and the holding of the breath out, (called *bāhya kumbhaka*, or 'BK'). This is a quite different (although related) understanding of this sūtra's meaning.

Each of these three interpretations has value and can provide a useful springboard for us to examine the question of seated breathing practices, but it is the first understanding that is the most favoured by Desikachar and his students.

The meaning of prāṇāyāma

What do we mean by prāṇāyāma? Practising movements or āsana with synchronised breathing is *not* prāṇāyāma: prāṇāyāma is the conscious use of the breath in a static seated position. Desikachar described the relationship between body and breath in āsana and prāṇāyāma thus: "In āsana, we use the breath to support the body; in prāṇāyāma, we use the body to support the breath".[1] In āsana our focus is on the body – the feelings that arise, the quality of the movement or the stretch, and the primary tool in refining the body's movements and stretching is the breath. Here, breath supports body. This is reversed in prāṇāyāma: now the body must simply remain still and comfortable, supporting the movements of the breath. This requires both stability and freedom in the vertical axis (the spine) and also in the horizontal axis (the hips, knees and ankles). Only then can the two great chambers of the torso, the chest and the abdomen, be free to move, expand and contract in a way the allows for the free passage of breath and thus the circulation of energy.

Prāṇāyāma is the final word of YS 2.49 and, as it is the key topic of this chapter, it's worth also exploring its component parts. It is made up of two words, *prāṇa* and *āyāma*. We have already seen how *prāṇa* can be understood as energy (akin to the Chinese concept of *chi* or *qi*). Desikachar often described *prāṇa* as "a friend of *puruṣa*": we can think of *prāṇa* as a sort of 'go-between' linking *puruṣa* and *prakṛti* and allowing them to function together.

The second word, *āyāma,* is often translated as 'extended' or 'stretched' – and many translate this sūtra along the lines of 'prāṇāyāma is the lengthening (*āyāma*) of the breath (*prāṇa*)'. But the prefix *ā* here also reverses the direction with regard to the subject, thus *āyāma* means 'to extend *inwards*' – to return, to come back. In the practice of prāṇāyāma, we are concentrating our dissipated energy (*prāṇa*) by extending it *inwards* and

1. Personal communication.

making it flow powerfully and deeply within us, and thereby centring ourselves.

Starting to practise prāṇāyāma

From a traditional Haṭha Yoga perspective, prāṇāyāma is *the* essential practice.[2] Whilst āsana is important, it is through the practice of prāṇāyāma that the yogi starts to manipulate the energies of the body and really turns inwards. It has its dangers, however. The *Haṭha Yoga Pradīpikā* has some serious warnings: "As the lion, elephant or tiger is tamed gradually, even so should *prāṇa* be brought under control, else it will kill the practitioner" (HYP 2.15). Perhaps it is for these reasons that prāṇāyāma is rarely taught in group yoga classes, and also less commonly practised. It can be viewed as an esoteric practice whereby one has to have mastered all the āsana before one is competent to practice prāṇāyāma.[3] But what does it mean to have mastered all the postures? For us, the prerequisite for prāṇāyāma practice is simply an ability to remain in a comfortable seated posture with the qualities of both *sthira* and *sukha*.

There are also other reasons why prāṇāyāma practice is often cursory, forgotten, or omitted. Prāṇāyāma is a subtler practice than āsana. A beginner can feel their hamstrings stretching, their hips opening or their back working. From the first class of āsana, a novice practitioner can notice a considerable difference in their mental outlook, a feeling of calm and focus. But prāṇāyāma is more challenging, and many people wonder what exactly they are doing with their breath (and why) – especially when it involves fiddling with the nostrils and counting! Paul Harvey used to say that āsana works "from the outside in" and is therefore more immediately noticeable, while prāṇāyāma works "from the inside out".[4] It takes time to feel its potency and its effects. Āsana also has many potential variations; there are endless ways that we can turn and move our bodies to make new shapes or sequences. In this sense, āsana can be fun,

2. Krishnamacharya was emphatic: *haṭha yoga* **is** prāṇāyāma.

3. BKS Iyengar compares āsana with undergraduate studies, whilst prāṇāyāma is postgraduate – it is an advanced practice.

4. Personal communication.

entertaining and engaging. But prāṇāyāma is a more 'naked practice'; although there are many different possibilities of practice, the parameters are much reduced, and they all basically require us to remain seated and still, and focus on the subtle variations we can make in the techniques of breathing.

The three viewing towers of prāṇāyāma

YS 2.50 bāhya-abhyantara-stambha-vṛttiḥ deśa-kāla-saṃkhyābhiḥ paridṛṣṭo dīrgha-sūkṣmaḥ

By observing the exhalation, the inhalation and the pauses between them from three perspectives (placing our attention, varying their relative lengths and considering the number of repetitions), we can refine both the length and subtlety of the whole breath[5]

Patañjali starts by identifying the three parts of the breath: *bāhya* (exhale), *abhyantara* (inhale) and *stambha-vṛttiḥ* (*kumbhaka*). There is an important order to this: the exhalation comes first and it is our primary concern because it is the foundation for the rest of the breath. As long as the exhalation is smooth, we can be assured that we are working within our limits. As Desikachar says:

> "Whichever technique we choose, the most important part of prāṇāyāma is the exhalation. If the quality of the exhalation is not good, the quality of the whole prāṇāyāma practice is adversely affected. When someone is not able to breathe out slowly and quietly it means that he or she is not ready for prāṇāyāma, either mentally or otherwise. Indeed, some texts give this warning: if the inhalation is rough we do not have to worry, but if the exhalation is uneven it is a sign of illness, either present or impending."[6]

5. This understanding of the three parts of the breath (exhalation, inhalation and pauses) is how this sūtra has been presented by students of Desikachar. Vyāsa uses the term *bāhya* to refer to the BK, the term *abhyantara* to refer to the AK, and the term *stambha-vṛtti* to refer 'suppression' (stopping) of the breath. See Hariharānanda, *Yoga Philosophy of Patañjali*, State University of New York Press, 1983, p. 234.

6. *Heart of Yoga*, p. 59.

Having identified the three different parts of the breath (the exhalation, *bāhya*; the inhalation, *abhyantara*; and the pauses between, *stambha vṛtti*), Patañjali gives us three 'viewing towers', from which we can gain a perspective on, and also some control over, our breath. These three are the essential variables of the breath and they define what we can do within prāṇāyāma practice:

- ***deśa*** – means 'place' and so this refers to where we focus our attention. Generally, this is seen as the primary site of breath control, the place where we create a valve to lengthen and refine the quality of the breath. Thus, in nostril control breathing, it would be in the nostril through which we are inhaling or exhaling; in *ujjāyī*, it is the throat; and in *śītalī* or *sītkārī*, it is the tongue. However, *deśa* can also refer to other places in the body where we might place our focus, for example, the chest as we inhale and the abdomen as we exhale.

- ***kāla*** – means 'time'. Here Patañjali is referring to the duration of the breath. This implies investigating how to make the breath long and the effects of its different components. An important technique for this is to formally explore the relative timings of the different parts of the breath – in other words, ratio. Although we never make the inhalation longer than the exhalation (this would be too stimulating), by making them equal, there is a mild *bṛṃhaṇa* quality which can be enhanced by adding a hold (AK) after the inhalation. Similarly, the longer we make the exhalation in relationship to the inhalation, the more we make the breath *laṅghana*. This can also be enhanced by the addition of a pause (BK) after the exhalation.

- ***saṃkhyā*** – the last parameter is that of numbers. *Sam* links to the English word 'sum' and *khyā*, in this context, is 'count'. *Saṃkhyā* thus refers to the total number of breaths we take. We may take six breaths with one ratio (as preparation), a further twelve breaths with a more intense ratio (as the main body of the practice) and finally six breaths of a lighter ratio as a 'cool down'. Therefore, *saṃkhyā* implies both the overall length of the practice, which in some measure at least determines its intensity, and its structure in terms of the *vinyāsa krama*, the number of breaths at each stage and their progression.

Patañjali uses the term *paridṛṣṭa* ('to view from all around') to refer to how we observe these three conditions. These are the watchtowers – three different perspectives on the breath from which we can lengthen and refine. This is a very important principle that Swami Hariharānanda[7] reminds us about in relation to *saṃyama* (meditative enquiry). He emphasises that to really understand something we must investigate it from different perspectives so that our comprehension is complete and 'well rounded'. Thus, *paridṛṣṭa* is a general and important principle in practice: to approach and investigate from all sides, with different supports and perspectives. Only when these three parameters have been sensitively observed and refined, do we move towards a breath with the ideal twin qualities of *dīrgha* (long) and *sūkṣma* (subtle).

At an initial level, *dīrgha* can simply imply a lengthening of the breath, and *sūkṣma* a refining of it, such that it becomes quiet, smooth and even. This is certainly an essential prerequisite, but as we develop our practice more deeply, we might reflect on more nuanced meanings. Simply lengthening the breath may be limited – like a stretched-out piece of chewing gum, as Peter Hersnack often used to say. *Dīrgha* is not necessarily simply 'more of the same'; instead, it is (to use Peter's words again) "where the breath opens up on itself to create timeless holes or pockets of infinity".[8] The very quality of the breath becomes more spacious. In the same way, we can think of *sūkṣma* not just as making the breath quieter – a change in volume, but rather a 'change in the frequency', in the actual quality as well.

Dīrgha and *sūkṣma* are the fruit of *deśa, kāla* and *saṃkhyā*. Because they are essential qualities of the breath

7. See Hariharānanda, op. cit. p. 253: "the object contemplated upon has to be thought of from all sides and in all its aspects..."

8. Personal communication.

in this practice, they are to prāṇāyāma what *sthira* and *sukha* are to āsana.

The three fruits of prāṇāyāma

YS 2.51 bāhya-abhyantara-viṣaya-ākṣepī caturthaḥ

In the fourth state (of breathing), the normal process of 'inhalation' and 'exhalation' are transcended

This is a mysterious sūtra. Wendy Doniger[9] discusses how there are many groups of three in the Indian philosophical tradition, and they are joined – and then transcended – by a mysterious fourth principle. The first three are worldly; the fourth is of another dimension. Thus, for example, in the four aims of life (*puruṣārtha)*, the first three – duty, the pursuit of wealth and sensual fulfilment (*dharma, artha and kāma* respectively) – belong to the world and apply to everyone all the time. The fourth one, liberation (*mokṣa*) is of a different order and will only be pursued by a limited number of people. Similarly, there are three stages to life (*āśrama*) for all normal people: student, householder and retired (*brahmacarya, gṛhastha* and *vanaprastha* respectively). But a fourth category, *saṃnyāsa*, suggests the possibility of a complete renunciation. There are even three strands which create the fabric of *prakṛti – tamas, rajas* and *sattva*. Thus, *prakṛti* is called *saguṇa* – with qualities. But beyond these is *puruṣa*, which is without qualities and therefore *nirguṇa*.

In this sūtra on prāṇāyāma, we are introduced to a mysterious fourth type of breath which is of a different order to anything to do with conscious inhalation, exhalation or the stopping of the breath. Desikachar rather cryptically comments, "An entirely different state of breathing appears in the state of yoga... It is not possible to be more specific."[10] It is easy to view this sūtra as something of an oddball – and so esoteric that it really has little relevance to

9. Wendy Doniger, *The Hindus: An Alternative History* (Penguin USA, 2009), pp. 199–211.

10. TKV Desikachar, *Patañjali's Yogasūtras* (Affiliated East-West Press Ltd, 1987).

us mere mortals. But if we view it as something reachable, real and fundamental to prāṇāyāma then it can have more relevance. We can see it as a type of breathing where volition and intention have been transcended, and the breath has become so subtle that concepts of 'inside' and 'outside' seem no longer to apply. The difference between inhalation, exhalation and pauses is barely perceptible: the breath (and by implication, the thoughts) become like 'ripples on the surface of Being'.[11] This new quality of the breath (and the mind), where there is hardly any movement, opens up a spaciousness *within the breath itself*. This space is a space for perception, for presence and for freedom. We can view all the techniques of prāṇāyāma (which are described in more detail below) as steps to move us towards this fourth type of breathing; they are platforms that we build and work with in order to leap off and fly freely. This fourth type of breathing is a sign that something has opened to the very source of the breath.

YS 2.52 tataḥ kṣiyate prakāśa-āvaraṇam

From this, blockages are destroyed and our inner light is revealed

Although it is not usual, we can consider this clear statement to be referring directly to YS 2.51, the previous sūtra (as opposed to YS 2.50). Thus: a state of clarity arises when our breath has become so subtle that a new quality of spaciousness has opened it up from inside. This state of clarity marks the fruition of a new type of breathing. The word *āvaraṇa* (covering) is a synonym for *tamas*;[12] and it is this *tamas*, which is said to obscure our vision and perception. Prāṇāyāma dissolves (*kṣiyate*) that which obscures (*tamas*). As the *tamas* is reduced, so our natural clarity is enhanced. Here Patañjali uses the word *prakāśa*, which as we have seen, refers to *sattva guṇa*. So, we have a direct statement about how the correct practice of prāṇāyāma reduces *tamas* and enhances both *sattva*

11. This phrase comes from Eckhart Tolle, and is the title of an interview with him by Andrew Cohen in *What is Enlightenment?* magazine, no 18, Fall/Winter 2000.

12. The essential quality of *tamas* is described as *varanakam* (enveloping, obscuring) in the *Sāṃkhya Kārikā* v.13.

and perception. Certainly, we are often more sensitive, clearer, and our eyes appear to sparkle, after prolonged and dedicated prāṇāyāma practice.

YS 2.53 dhāraṇāsu ca yogyatā manasaḥ

And the mind is made fit for dhāraṇā

Dhāraṇā is the doorway into meditation, and it requires us to stay with one thought, or object, for a length of time. In other words, *dhāraṇā* requires a certain stability of mind: we can't focus on a single principle if we are distracted. In this final fruit of prāṇāyāma, Patañjali gives us another compelling reason to practice: it reduces movement (*rajas*) and thus agitation in the mind and senses.[13] Anyone who has developed their prāṇāyāma practice will know that the ability to sit still for meditative practices is hugely enhanced by some seated breathing; it is as if prāṇāyāma has prepared the ground and now *dhāraṇā* can begin to arise with much less effort. Interestingly, Patañjali uses the suffix *su* at the end of *dhāraṇā*. *Su* implies a plural – many forms of *dhāraṇā* can arise. In Chapter 3 of the Yoga Sūtra (*Vibhūti Pāda*), Patañjali describes the possibilities of directing the mind towards many different objects, and explores the various sorts of powers (*siddhi*) which arise from such practices.

13. Often when comparing āsana and prāṇāyāma, āsana is seen as remedy for excess *rajas* and prāṇāyāma as a remedy for excess *tamas* in the mind. This is certainly the teaching of Krishnamacharya's student Srivatsa Ramaswami. However, this is something of a generalisation and actually prāṇāyāma itself can work on both of these problematic *guṇa* to prepare for meditation.

Sādhana: Techniques of prāṇāyāma

As with āsana, Patañjali has very little to say in the Yoga Sūtra about the actual mechanics of practicing prāṇāyāma. Later Haṭha Yoga texts have much more information on the different techniques – their application, their value and their potential dangers. The *Haṭha Yoga Pradīpikā* presents *nāḍī śodhana* as the definitive prāṇāyāma technique.[14] It lists a further eight techniques which are collectively called

14. See HYP 2.7–21.

kumbhaka.[15] These are *sūrya bhedana, ujjāyī, sītkārī, śītalī, bhastrikā, bhrāmarī, mūrcchā* and *plāvinī*. Another common technique practiced in yoga classes is *kapālabhāti,* but this is described as a *kriyā*[16] (cleansing action) in the HYP. While we regularly use *ujjāyī, sītkārī, śītalī* and sometimes *sūrya bhedana, bhastrikā* and *bhrāmarī,* it is unusual to practise *mūrcchā* and *plāvinī*. Krishnamacharya, and then subsequently his students, added some additional techniques to this list: *anuloma ujjāyī, viloma ujjāyī* and *pratiloma ujjāyī*. These additions are basically modifications of *nāḍī śodhana* using *ujjāyī* to punctuate the rhythm of the nostril control. Each has a role in helping us to access *nāḍī śodhana*; however, to view them as only training techniques is to undervalue their unique flavours. Particularly when combined with creative *bhāvana*, they can each lead to unique experiences and contribute to the *paridṛṣṭa* of the breath, or support therapeutic goals.

The first watchtower: *Deśa* – placing of the attention

The 'placing of the attention' is a way that we can understand two aspects of prāṇāyāma: *bhāvana* and also the actual technique. The use of *bhāvana* can be particularly powerful when working with prāṇāyāma; it transforms a simple breathing practice into one which profoundly engages the mind. Each inhalation can invite a sense of opening from the inside, whilst each exhalation can invite a feeling of the breath withdrawing. We can also visualise something of the difference between left and right – the left linking to the lunar channel and qualities of coolness and the feminine, whilst the right side links to the solar channel, heat and the masculine. By 'placing our attention' in this way, we deepen our involvement and put something of ourselves into the practice.

The second aspect, the 'placing of the attention with regard to technique', also transforms a simple practice. Just as we can

15. See HYP 2.48–70 for more detail on these techniques. Some teachers consider the distinction between *nāḍī śodhana* and the other techniques classified as *kumbhaka* as very significant, as if *nāḍī śodhana* is the only real prāṇāyāma. Others take *kumbhaka* just as a word to refer to different techniques. This was Krishnamacharya's view: the other techniques are still prāṇāyāma, but *nāḍī śodhana* is the preeminent prāṇāyāma technique.

16. The word *kriyā* literally means 'action', but in the HYP it is understood to mean a purification technique. A common confusion is to equate the *kriyā* of haṭha yoga with the *kriyā yoga* of Patañjali's Yoga Sūtra.

divide āsana into various groups depending on the action of the spine,[17] so can we divide prāṇāyāma techniques into groups according to their primary place of regulation – nostril control, throat control or mouth control.

The support of the throat: *Ujjāyī*

We have already discussed *ujjāyī* in Chapter 9, but there is a subtle difference between how we use *ujjāyī* in āsana and in prāṇāyāma. In the former, it is usually a little louder (generally speaking, the more demanding the physical work, the louder the breath). In the latter, *ujjāyī* can be refined so that it is much more of a 'caress' of the throat – a gentle feeling, like silk on marble, and barely audible at all. *Ujjāyī* is a technique intimately linked to the body – it 'gives body to the breath'. However, we can over-control it and it becomes laboured and regimented. As we inhale, we may experience a profound opening from within. If, as we exhale, we can maintain this feeling, there is a feeling of the body remaining open as the breath 'withdraws' back to its source at our centre.

The breath, the spine, the chest and the abdomen are all brought in to play. When they are working harmoniously, the quality of *ujjāyī* becomes an *expression* of what is happening in the body, rather than as something manipulated, manufactured and controlled. *Ujjāyī* is thus a 'whole body' practice, not just something which happens in the throat. Nevertheless, it is still necessary to apply the restriction in the throat to create the friction required for *ujjāyī*.

The support of the nostrils: Nostril control breathing

Implicit in the technique of *ujjāyī* is a vertical polarity – that of head and pelvis, of chest and abdomen, and *prāṇa* and *apāna*. But it's also worth remembering that *ujjāyī* is

17. For example, forward bends, backward bends, twists and lateral flexion.

fundamentally a symmetrical technique; it does not address the relationship between the two sides of the body. It is only when we introduce nostril control breathing that the breath becomes asymmetrical. While *ujjāyī* is unifying, we could say the introduction of nostril control breathing is separating. It allows us to view one side from the other side, to make distinctions – and thereby to forge new relationships between left and right. The hand position that enables nostril control breathing is *mṛgi mudrā* (fig 10.1).

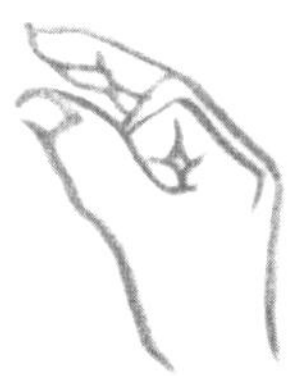

fig 10.1

Mṛgi mudrā allows us to create a very fine valve in the nostril to regulate the breath. Whether one is inhaling or exhaling, during alternate nostril breathing, one nostril is completely closed and the other is partially restricted.[18] The amount of pressure that we apply to the nostril through which we breathe will vary: if our nostril is completely clear, we may nearly completely close the nostril; if our nostril is less clear, it may be necessary to hardly close it at all. It is very important that no trace of *ujjāyī* remains as we breathe through one nostril – the throat should be completely relaxed and any noise or friction is experienced only in the nostril. The nostril, therefore, is the *deśa*.

Ujjāyī is a great technique for use in āsana, but undoubtedly it is less subtle than nostril control breathing. By closing one nostril completely, and then partially closing the other, we are in effect significantly reducing the area though which we breathe with the aim of refining the breath. Because of this significant reduction, if there is any blockage, people can easily feel claustrophobic with these techniques. Refining the breath is important, but another

18. This detail, partial restriction of the nostril through which you are breathing, is crucial and is commonly overlooked or misunderstood.

key difference between *ujjāyī* and nostril control is that *ujjāyī* is more linked to the body, whereas nostril control is more linked to the mind. The experience of the breath is more downwards (and into the body) with *ujjāyī*, and more upwards (and into the head) with nostril control techniques.

By introducing nostril breathing at various points in the breathing cycle, the following three variations of *ujjāyī* allow us to move towards *nāḍī śodhana.*[19]

Anuloma Ujjāyī: Bringing the body into presence

The first nostril control technique that we introduce is *anuloma ujjāyī* – literally 'with the grain of the hair' (*anu* means 'with', *loman* is hair). Because the hairs in the nostrils point towards the opening, they act as a filter to inhaled air. Going with the grain, therefore, is moving outwards and it is linked to the exhalation. *Anuloma ujjāyī* uses *ujjāyī* (the throat) to modulate and support the breath on the inhalation, but transfers that support to one nostril as we exhale. The *deśa* thus shifts: throat as we inhale, one nostril as we exhale.

Anuloma ujjāyī is a tool for refining and lengthening the exhalation, and it helps to clear the nostrils. Because it favours lengthening the exhalation it is often thought of as a *laṅghana* technique, and a relaxing prāṇāyāma.

Because *ujjāyī* links more to the body, and nostril control more to mind, we can also understand *anuloma ujjāyī* as applying *ujjāyī* on the inhalation (body focus), and nostril control on the exhalation (mental focus). Thus *anuloma ujjāyī* "allows the mind (nostril control on exhale) to take support on the body (*ujjāyī* on inhale)".[20] In this way, the practice of *anuloma ujjāyī* reveals something about our current bodily state; the body comes into presence. Students sometimes say that *anuloma ujjāyī* leaves them feeling tired and that it is too *laṅghana*. But if we understand the technique as *becoming present to the state of the body*, then

19. As well as being variations of *ujjāyī*, they could be seen as modifications of *nāḍī śodhana*, since they involve a combination of using both *ujjāyī* and nostril control.

20. Peter Hersnack presented this way of working on numerous workshops and retreats.

actually they are simply realising how tired they are; their bodily state is revealed. The body is brought into presence.

Viloma Ujjāyī: Allowing the mind to become a support for the body

Viloma ujjāyī is the opposite of *anuloma ujjāyī*.[21] *Vi* used here as a prefix means 'against' – so this technique is 'against the grain of the hair'. In *viloma ujjāyī,* we inhale through a single nostril and exhale through both using *ujjāyī.* The *deśa* moves from the nostril (on the inhalation) to the throat (on the exhalation). Because the nostril is a conical shape, with the widest part at the entrance, when we inhale we are breathing into a narrowing space. By only inhaling into one nostril and then by adding a further restriction using *mṛgi mudrā,* this technique can feel quite suffocating to the novice. However, to a more experienced practitioner, the friction caused by the *mṛgi mudrā* on the inhalation can really support the refinement and lengthening of the inhalation. Moreover, *viloma ujjāyī* allows "the mind (nostril control on inhale) to become a support for the body (*ujjāyī* on exhale)".[22] Thus, it helps us to actualise and to embody – by translating ideas and thoughts into bodily possibilities. In other words, it helps us to get things done.

Pratiloma Ujjāyī: Giving us a stable presence in the world

The final technique lies somewhere between *ujjāyī* and *nāḍī śodhana,* and is a combination of the *anuloma* and *viloma ujjāyī* described above. We breathe in using *ujjāyī,* we exhale through the left nostril (*anuloma ujjāyī*), and then we breathe in though the left and exhale using *ujjāyī* (*viloma ujjāyī*). This pattern is then repeated on the right side. In *pratiloma ujjāyī,* the *deśa* shifts after every inhale. We move from the throat to one nostril, back to the throat and then to the other nostril. The technique neither favours the inhalation

21. Srivatsa Ramaswami, another of Krishnamacharya's students, calls this technique *pratiloma*; what we describe here as *pratiloma,* he calls *viloma*. It's probably not worth getting too concerned about which is correct – the main thing is we are in agreement about the techniques, rather than their names!

22. Peter Hersnack, personal communication.

nor the exhalation; it is 'the Great Equaliser'. It requires us to remain present and focused; the continuous change of *deśa* demands our involvement. Peter Hersnack said of this technique that it "gives us a stable presence in the world".[23] *Pratiloma ujjāyī* is certainly a very engaging technique; it has something of everything and the throat breathing provides a sort of 'release valve' for any tension accrued during nostril control. This is excellent preparation for meditative practices and also for developing inhalations, exhalations and *kumbhaka* evenly.

Nāḍī śodhana: Giving us an active presence in the world

The prāṇāyāma technique *par excellence* is *nāḍī śodhana. Nāḍī* means 'channel' or 'river', whilst *śodhana* is a means of cleansing (*śauca*); so *nāḍī śodhana* is the technique that purifies the channels through which our *prāṇa* runs. This is nostril control with no compromise: we inhale through the left nostril and then exhale through the right; this is then reversed so we inhale through the right and exhale through the left. There is no trace of *ujjāyī*; the friction of the breath is felt entirely in the nostrils and so the *deśa* simply moves from one nostril to the other.

In Haṭha Yoga's esoteric conception of the energetic body, the two nostrils symbolise an important polarity. The left nostril (*iḍā*) is associated with the feminine, the moon and with cooling, while the right nostril (*piṅgalā*) is associated with the masculine, the sun and heating. When we breathe through the left nostril, our *prāṇa* is said to flow in *iḍā nāḍī*, likewise breathing though the right nostril means it flows in *piṅgalā nāḍī*. These two great channels weave their way down the vertical axis, intersecting at highly charged points known as *cakra* (fig 10.2).

It is said that as long as we remain caught in the duality of male/female or sun/moon, then we remain, at some level, divided from the world and ourselves. We are cut off,

23. Personal communication.

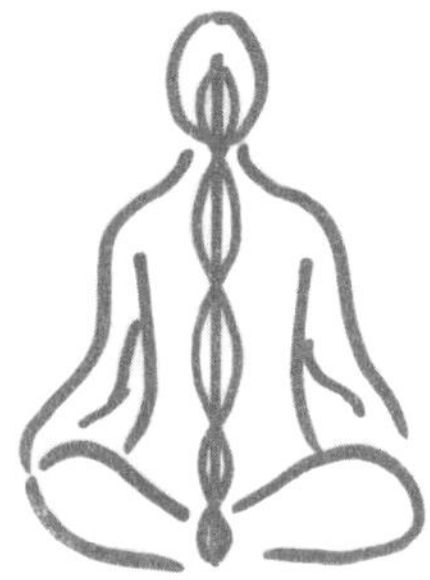

fig 10.2

and we experience isolation. The project of Haṭha Yoga is to bring these two aspects into a harmonious relationship that facilitates an experience of true presence, of Being There, undivided. Symbolically, this is described as the breath flowing in the (usually blocked) central channel – the *suṣumṇā* – and *nāḍī śodhana* is the practice to facilitate this.

An effective *bhāvana* which Peter Hersnack sometimes taught involved a gentle lifting on one side of the abdomen as we exhale through one nostril (on the same side as the lift), and a 'placing down' on the same side as we inhale. He called this 'an inner walk'. This 'inner walk' is also a sort of 'inner dialogue' between our two sides and it creates both stability and openness. *Nāḍī śodhana* thus gives us, in Peter's words, "an active presence in the world."[24]

The support of the mouth/tongue

In the following two prāṇāyāma techniques, the *deśa* is placed in the mouth – and specifically the tongue – as we inhale.

Śītalī: The cooling breath

This technique requires us to curl the tongue into a tube and stick it out as we breathe in, 'drinking' the air in, as if through a straw. At the same time, we lift the chin as if drinking from a glass making the inhalation as quiet and smooth as possible. At the end of the inhalation, we then

24. Personal communication.

retract the tongue and close the mouth, lift the tongue to the palate, and lower the chin back down to stabilise the head before finally exhaling slowly using *ujjāyī*. Implicit in the technique, therefore, is a short pause after the inhalation. Because the inhaled air travels through the tube of the tongue, it picks up moisture and the breath feels refreshing and cool as it enters the system, which is why *śītalī* is known as 'the cooling breath'. It is very important to reconnect the tongue to the roof of the mouth after inhalation because this stimulates salivation and keeps the tongue moist; if we don't, then after a few breaths the tongue begins to feel like a dried-out piece of leather in the mouth. As an interesting variation to engage us, and refine the exhalation and to prepare for further techniques involving the nostrils, *śītalī* can also be combined with alternative nostril breathing exhalation.

It is best used sparingly – probably no more than about twelve breaths at a time. However, it can be an excellent therapeutic tool; it soothes any tendency towards nausea, heartburn or indigestion, as well as calming the mind. It is a very useful to combine *śītalī* with other techniques (for example, *anuloma ujjāyī* or *nāḍī śodhana*) in a longer prāṇāyāma practice.

Finally, it is also a technique that can effectively be used in āsana – for example in *mahā mudrā*, in the cat (*cakravākāsana*) and even in the headstand (*śirṣāsana*) – although obviously here there would be no movement of the head.

Of course, not everyone can actually roll their tongue in such a way that makes *śītalī* possible and in such cases, we use *sītkārī*. Although the *Haṭha Yoga Pradīpikā* describes it as a completely different technique, we use *sītkārī* as a modification for those who are unable to practice *śītalī*.

Sītkārī: The hissing breath

Rather charmingly, the *Haṭha Yoga Pradīpikā* claims that the diligent practitioner of *sītkārī* will become "a second God of

Love" (HYP 2.54). As with *śītalī* the breath is inhaled through the mouth, the difference being that instead of drawing the breath through the curled tongue, here the tongue is pressed against the lower teeth (with the tip pointing downwards) and the breath drawn over the tongue. This creates a slight hissing sound (*sītkārī* literally means 'creating a "*ssss*" sound'). The tongue also needs to be re-moisturised using *sītkārī* for the same reasons as *śītalī*. In fact, most of what can be said of *śītalī* can also apply to *sītkārī*.

The first watchtower: Summary

Although we have not addressed some of the prāṇāyāmas referred to in the *Haṭha Yoga Pradīpikā,* the above comprise the most common techniques we practise. We can see how we have three major *deśa* for the attention (throat, nostrils and mouth) in five possible combinations:

- Throat: *ujjāyī*
- Throat and nostril: *anuloma ujjāyī, viloma ujjāyī* and *pratiloma ujjāyī*
- Nostril*: nāḍī śodhana*
- Mouth and throat: *śītalī* or *sītkārī* with *ujjāyī* on exhale
- Mouth and nostril: *śītalī* or *sītkārī* with nostril control on exhale

The second watchtower: *Kāla* – the length of the breath

The second means to gain perspective on the breath is by regulating its rhythm. By dividing the breath into four parts and then consciously adjusting their various lengths in relationship to one another, we can alter both the feeling and the effect of the prāṇāyāma technique considerably. We can make the breath more stimulating by giving more proportional length to the inhalation and *antaḥ kumbhaka* (AK), or we could make the breath more relaxing by emphasising the exhalation and *bāhya kumbhaka* (BK).

Traditionally, the rhythms were broadly divided into two categories: *samavṛtti* and *viṣamavṛtti*. In *samavṛtti*, the separate parts of the breath are equal in length:

in	AK	ex	BK
1	1	1	1

If we make each unit 4 seconds, we would have one breath cycle lasting 16 seconds. This is very different from making each unit 12 seconds and having a 48-second complete breath. Both are *samavṛtti*, but the longer breath is obviously far more intense and demanding. Thus, the length (of the complete breath) as well as the rhythm, are significant factors in defining intensity.

Strictly speaking, all other rhythms are *viṣamavṛtti*, that is, having unequal parts. However, by dropping the lengths of the AK and the BK equally (or indeed, excluding them altogether), we can experience a 'modified' *samavṛtti*, a sort of '*samavṛtti* light':

in	AK	ex	BK
1	½	1	½
or			
1	0	1	0

Both of these are very effective rhythms to produce a feeling of containment and stability. In fact, because these are less intense than a full 1.1.1.1 rhythm, they have a more balanced feel to them; 1.1.1.1 can be very demanding!

There is a huge variety of potential *viṣamavṛtti* rhythms, and their spectrum can be from the very mild and therapeutic to the extremely intense. We should adhere to a few general principles for safety's sake (these apply to *samavṛtti* rhythms too):

- The breath should always remain smooth and undisturbed – ragged or broken breaths are an indication that we have gone too far and need to shorten the complete length or modify the rhythm.

- The quality of the exhalation is paramount whereas a little compromise in the quality of the inhalation is okay. The exhalation is the real litmus test.
- The length of the inhalation should never be greater than the exhalation. A natural breath has a slightly longer exhalation than inhalation, so by making them equal we are already favouring the inhalation a little. To consciously make the inhalation longer disturbs the overall balance and is over-stimulating.
- Although the inhalation should not be longer than the exhalation, the combined length of the inhalation and the AK may be longer than the exhalation. Thus 1.1.1.0 is fine, whereas 2.0.1.0 is not.

What are we looking for when practicing *viṣamavṛtti* prāṇāyāma? Do we want a more *laṅghana* or more *bṛṃhaṇa* effect? The specific technique, the length of the breath and its rhythm will all have a bearing on this. A longer complete breath length will *tend* to exaggerate the rhythm's intrinsic effect.

Any rhythm that favours the inhalation and AK over the exhalation and BK is *bṛṃhaṇa*. Common *bṛṃhaṇa* rhythms might include:

1	½	1	0
1	1	1	0
1	2	1	0
1	4	2	0[25]

If we want to make the breath more *laṅghana,* we work with cultivating the exhalation and then the BK. Common *laṅghana* examples include:

1	0	1½	0
1	0	2	0
1	0	1½	½
1	0	2	1

25. Although this last rhythm is presented in the HYP, we would be cautious with its application. Such a long AK requires considerable training, and can lead to disturbance and irritability.

Some people, it has to be said, loathe counting their breath. And when we use a metronome – as we often do – they feel 'boxed in'. It is very important therefore, to go into these sorts of practices with an open attitude, to embrace the counting as a *support* rather than as a prison. Counting can help us to keep focused, it can function as a mirror, and it can be a precision tool for refining and training our breath. It is easy to simply drift off into vague meanderings with the breath if one doesn't count; the rhythm gives the prāṇāyāma a crispness, a structure and an intensity which may otherwise be lost. For some, an alternative form of counting is to practice with a mantra – repeating the mantra perhaps once on the inhalation and twice on the exhalation (this would be a *laṅghana* rhythm). This type of prāṇāyāma is called *samantraka* (literally 'with mantra') and it is very effective.

The major issue with regard to *kāla* in prāṇāyāma is that of over-control. The pre-ordained rhythms can sometimes constrain the breath (and the mind) and the breath then becomes regimented and 'audited'. The ideal is to count the breath without overly influencing it, to let it retain its innocence. We need to observe the breath without judgement, give it the freedom to play a little and to surprise us. It's a fine line to walk.

The third watchtower: *Saṃkhyā* – numbering the breath

The final point of observation for the breath is *saṃkhyā*, number. It may seem trivial or overstated, but simply counting the number of breaths we take is one more important tool in refining and developing our practice. The minimum length for a prāṇāyāma practice is twelve breaths; anything less is hardly sufficient. By using our thumb as a marker, we can conveniently count these twelve breaths on the inside of our fingers (fig 10.3).

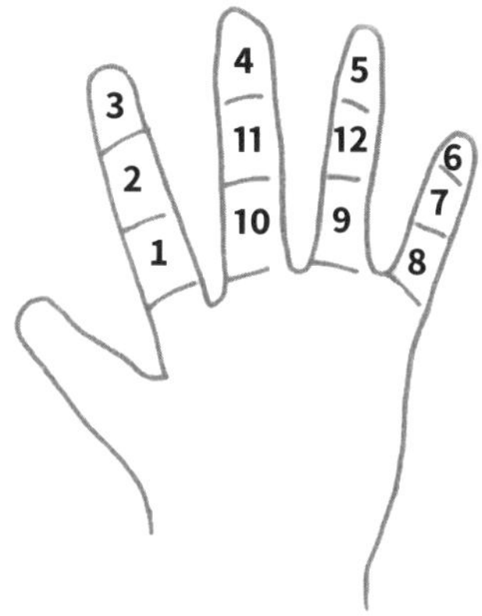

fig 10.3

Building longer practices usually involves a *vinyāsa krama,* so that we increase the intensity of the breath until we reach the goal, and then we step back down to complete the practice. A moderate practice would be 18–30 breaths, whereas a more intense practice might be 40 breaths or longer.

The way we increase the intensity could involve developing either the technique or the rhythm, or indeed, both. However, unless we are experienced practitioners who know our breath well, it is generally advisable to only change one variable at a time (either the technique, the length or the rhythm) as we progress towards our goal. When we build up a practice in this way, we would suggest a minimum count of four breaths (although more commonly six breaths) at each step. It is common to maintain the peak of the practice for twelve breaths – this shows a level of mastery at a particular ratio. It is possible to 'fake' six breaths or less, but twelve breaths will show if we have exceeded our capacity.

Below are three examples of *vinyāsa krama* in prāṇāyāma using *saṃkhyā*. In the first, there is a development of technique, in the second a development of rhythm, and finally, a development of both. It is important to understand that these are three examples out of many possible structures and they are not to be taken as iconic or definitive.

In each, the *saṃkhyā*, or number of breaths at each stage, provides a framing structure.

Development of technique (*deśa*)

Here we start with six breaths of *ujjāyī* to establish a basic breath length. Then we add a further six breaths of nostril control on the exhalation (*anuloma ujjāyī*) to help clear the nostrils as a preparation for the goal of *nāḍī śodhana*. We maintain our goal for twelve breaths at the peak of the practice. Then we descend in two steps, returning to *ujjāyī* before finally letting the breath be free for a few breaths. The complete practice is 30 breaths long, making it a moderately long practice.

	***deśa* (place)**	***kāla* (rhythm)**	***saṃkhyā* (number)**
Preparation	*ujjāyī* (throat)	free	6 breaths
Intensification	*anuloma ujjāyī* (throat and nostril)	free	6 breaths
Goal	*nāḍī śodhana* (nostril)	free	12 breaths
Descent	*ujjāyī* (throat)	free	4 breaths
Reintegration	free	free	4+ breaths

Development of rhythm (*kāla*)

In this second example of a *vinyāsa krama,* we intensify the rhythm. We start with *anuloma ujjāyī* to establish a good breath length for six breaths, and here we make the exhalation and the inhalation equal. We then increase the exhalation first for another six breaths (remember, the quality of the exhalation is always the key aspect to establish, and is the most important part of the breath). We then reach the goal of an exhalation which is twice as long as the inhalation and we maintain this for twelve breaths, as the main body of the practice. Having completed twelve breaths here, we drop back to a gentle *ujjāyī* and finish with some free breathing again.

	deśa (place)	*kāla* (rhythm)	*saṃkhyā* (number)
Preparation	*anuloma ujjāyī* (throat and nostril)	1 0 1 0	6 breaths
Intensification	*anuloma ujjāyī* (throat and nostril)	1 0 1½ 0	6 breaths
Goal	*anuloma ujjāyī* (throat and nostril)	1 0 2 0	12 breaths
Descent	*ujjāyī* (throat)	½ 0 1 0	4 breaths
Reintegration	free	free	4+ breaths

Development of technique (*deśa*) and rhythm (*kāla*)

In the final, slightly more complex example, we start with *śītalī* before introducing a further six breaths with the same rhythm of *anuloma ujjāyī,* and then six breaths of *nāḍī śodhana.* Staying with the same technique, we now intensify the rhythm by adding *kumbhaka* after both the inhale and the exhale and maintaining this for twelve breaths. Finally, we drop down again in two steps, first by coming to *ujjāyī* for four breaths with a lighter rhythm, and finally again letting the breath be free.

	deśa (place)	*kāla* (rhythm)	*saṃkhyā* (number)
Preparation	*sītalī* (mouth and throat)	1 0 1½ 0	6 breaths
Intensification 1	*anuloma ujjāyī* (throat and nostril)	1 0 1½ 0	6 breaths
Intensification 2	*nāḍī śodhana* (nostril)	1 0 1½ 0	6 breaths
Goal	*nāḍī śodhana* (nostril)	1 ½ 1½ ½	12 breaths
Descent	*ujjāyī* (throat and nostril)	½ 0 1 0	4 breaths
Reintegration	free	free	4+ breaths

In all three of these examples, you may notice a radical difference in the quality of the breath and also of the mind by the end of the practice. Having maintained a thorough, rigorous – and gentle – focus on the breath through the application of *deśa, kāla* and *saṃkhyā,* we can very easily move into more meditative practices where there is no control of the breath and the mind is settled.

Chapter 11

अहिंसासत्यास्तेयब्रह्मचर्यापरिग्रहा यमाः ।

Living with Others

YS 2.30 ahiṃsā-satya-asteya-brahmacarya-aparigrahāḥ yamāḥ

The five yama are non-violence, truthfulness, not-stealing, maintaining priorities and non-grasping

The *yama* are the first of the eight limbs of yoga (*aṣṭāṅga*), presented in the second chapter of the Yoga Sūtra. They are five attitudes, or (literally) restraints, suggested by Patañjali to free our relationships with others. Together, they create the conditions needed to establish a relationship and allow it to deepen in healthy ways by setting certain boundaries. Furthermore, they bring insights to relationships that take us towards a universal wisdom that goes beyond any specific relationship.

Desikachar often emphasised that yoga is relationship, and that the measure of our yoga practice lies in the quality of our relationships with the people around us. As we have seen, inherent in the word 'yoga' is the idea of the relationship between two separate principles. Such a relationship is profound, dynamic and respects the independence and fundamental differences between the two principles. This is a model that can also be applied to our interpersonal relationships where the two principles are ourselves and another person.

The *yama* are simply listed in YS 2.30. There follows an additional sūtra outlining the results as each *yama* is mastered and put into practice. Examining the fruits gives insight into what practising each *yama* might require.

When approaching the *yama* from a Western cultural perspective, it is easy to see them as moral commands that make us 'good' people. This can bring a sense of guilt or failure when we don't act well, or a tendency towards denial about our shortcomings. The approach of the Yoga Sūtra is eminently practical: cultivating the *yama* leads us towards greater freedom and clarity in our relationships. Furthermore, the *yama* are just one of the limbs of yoga to be practised, and 'practise' itself implies that we are in training and therefore not perfect. Perfection is, in this sense, less of a state than a direction.

Yoga requires disciplined practice, deep reflection and humility; embodying the *yama* requires the same. Fundamentally, we all need to live our own yoga, and to relate to those around us, as honestly and authentically as possible.

Self and other

The *yama* are conventionally presented as five attitudes or virtues to be adopted as ethical principles. They set boundaries on our behaviour. We can think of them as radiating from our centre towards others.

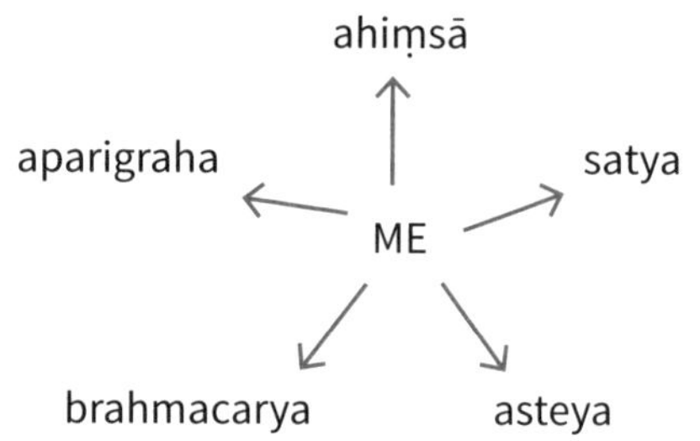

However, although it is true that the *yama* are qualities that we are trying to cultivate within ourselves, it is more helpful to understand them as applying to how we participate in our relationships.

ME	→	*ahiṃsā*	→	OTHER
ME	→	*satya*	→	OTHER
ME	→	*asteya*	→	OTHER
ME	→	*brahmacarya*	→	OTHER
ME	→	*aparigraha*	→	OTHER

We can divide them into two pairs, with the fifth *yama*, non-grasping (*aparigraha*), as the fruit of the others. The first pair, non-violence (*ahiṃsā*) and truthfulness (*satya*), establishes the basis of a relationship; *ahiṃsā* concerns the space that we can offer another person, and *satya* our participation in the relationship. The second pair, not stealing (*asteya*) and maintaining our priorities (*brahmacarya*), explains how the relationship can deepen without becoming cluttered with unnecessary baggage. Here, also, *asteya* is more concerned with the other person and *brahmacarya* more with our participation. The last term, *aparigraha*, allows us to go deeper in order to discover truths that take us beyond any individual relationship.

In this way, we can further define the *yama* as follows:

	Our impact on the other person	**Our part in the relationship**
Establishing the basis for the relationship	*ahiṃsā* Allowing space for the other person to be as they are	*satya* Being present and authentic
Deepening the relationship	*asteya* Not taking advantage of the other	*brahmacarya* Maintaining our priorities
Going beyond the relationship	*aparigraha* Non-accumulation in the relationship	

Establishing the basis: *ahiṃsā* and *satya*

YS 2.35 ahiṃsā-pratiṣṭhāyāṃ tat-sannidhau vaira-tyāgaḥ

In the presence of one established in non-violence, hostility diminishes

Ahiṃsā is literally 'non-violence' and is common to all the spiritual disciplines of India (and indeed the world). As the first *yama*, *ahiṃsā* is considered to be the foundation of the others – the rest should all be consistent with it and qualified by it. In some commentaries, the other *yama* are considered to be simply ways of strengthening and purifying *ahiṃsā* within us. *Ahiṃsā* is practised at the levels of body, speech and mind. In other words, it is not only about physical action, but also how we communicate with, and even how we think about, another person.

In YS 2.35, it is said that hostility is abandoned in the vicinity of one who has mastered *ahiṃsā*. If your personal space is threatened, it is easy to become defensive; if there is no perceived threat, there is no need to be defensive. In light of YS 2.35, we could reframe *ahiṃsā* as concerning the space that we offer the other person such that the impulse to be defensive does not arise. Non-violence in this sense means creating the conditions within a relationship for the other to simply be as they are, fully accepted, and valued, with no desire on our part to change them. So often in relationships, particularly as they become more established or involve loved ones, it is easy for the agenda of change to creep in: "If only he/she would be more....". If we understand *ahiṃsā* in this way its scope is expanded. Non-violence in a physical sense may be relatively easy to observe in our culture, but offering a non-judgemental space of acceptance to others is a constant challenge.

A relationship of yoga implies space; *saṃyoga* implies lack of space. We cannot practise *ahiṃsā* without giving the other both the space to communicate and the privilege of being heard. If we cannot offer another these, how can there be a genuine relationship?[1] The great peacemakers of history have always been willing to give their adversaries the space to be heard without feeling judged or threatened. In such a space, it is easy to let go of hostility and this forms the basis for real dialogue and the possibility of lasting peace. There are also many stories of yogis who lived in the forests and around whom wild creatures display no fear. Whether we call this an aura, 'vibe' or simply the atmosphere, animals seem intuitively sensitive to the quality of the space that surrounds individuals, just as the air seems charged with aggression that emanates from an angry or violent person.

Hiṃsā (violence, the opposite of *ahiṃsā*) begins with negative judgements about people. These often surface before any real contact or communication has taken place. Noticing the assumptions and judgements we make about people can be the starting point in developing a more open and accepting attitude to the world.

1. In the 1960s the famous psychotherapist Carl Rogers realised through his research the value for clients of really being listened to and heard. In this way, he validated the therapeutic power of *ahiṃsā*.

YS 2.36 satya-pratiṣṭhāyāṃ kriyā-phala āśrayatvam

When established in truthfulness, words and actions are consistent

Next, we come to *satya*, related to the Sanskrit term *sat,* meaning 'that which is real'. *Satya* is communication that reflects what is real or true, and is genuine and authentic. If *ahiṃsā* concerns the space that we can offer another in a relationship, *satya* is about the space that we occupy and the quality of the presence that we ourselves offer. *Satya* is concerned with our authenticity in the relationship, in being present, engaged and honest in our communication.

The first step in this is to be present, to put something of ourselves into the relationship, rather than hide behind some convenient mask. The second step is to communicate our truth rather than take refuge in superficial pleasantries. This is about authenticity, where there is congruence between our being and what we express. In stating our truth, however, there are limits. In counselling, we talk about 'appropriate transparency': that is, communicating honestly but bounded by a measure of appropriateness. What is this level of appropriateness? The *Mahābhārata* says, "Speak the truth which is pleasant. Do not speak unpleasant truths. Do not lie, even if the lies are pleasing to the ear." *Satya,* in other words, is always tempered by *ahiṃsā* and should never arise from anger, frustration or a wish to harm the other person.

We should also remember that **our** truth is not necessarily The Truth. The *Bṛhadāraṇyaka Upaniṣad* breaks down the word into three parts: *sa*, *ti* and *ya*: "The first and last syllables are the truth. In the middle is untruth. This untruth is enclosed on both sides by truth; thus truth prevails. Untruth does not hurt him who knows this." [2] In other words, our own partial or relative truth – truth with a small 't' if you like – is part of and contained by the larger, universal Truth. In the Yoga Sūtra this 'eternal truth' is called *ṛta*. In a practical sense, *ahiṃsā* and *satya* provide mutual

2. Bṛhadāraṇyaka Upaniṣad Chapter 5, section 5 verse 1

limits to the empathic space that we can offer to another and the appropriately transparent expression of our truth.

When we express ourselves truthfully and appropriately, there is an energetic power to which those around us and the world itself seem to respond. YS 2.36 states that when we are established in *satya*, there is a positive correspondence between our actions and their intended consequences. It is as if our words and actions have power because they reflect something inherently true. Those around us recognise this, and respond accordingly.

The space of *ahiṃsā* invites the other to feel accepted, their communication truly heard, with no need for defensiveness. The space of *satya* invites us to be authentically present and to communicate honestly and transparently, within the limits set by the principles of *ahiṃsā* and *satya* themselves. In such circumstances, the relationship may deepen, and the next pair of *yama* become more acutely relevant.

Keeping a relationship simple and open: *asteya* and *brahmacarya*

YS 2.37 asteya-pratiṣṭhāyāṃ sarva-ratna upasthānam

When established in not stealing, many treasures arise

As time passes in any relationship, things get more complicated. Perhaps we get to know someone better, we know more about their lives, and our interaction may become increasingly habitual. In couples, individuals can lose their independent identity outside of the relationship. What may have started as a relationship with clear boundaries, such as a working or professional relationship, can easily begin to overflow into other areas. Subtly, people can begin to manipulate or take advantage of one another, even if this happens on an entirely unconscious level. Familiarity, as the saying goes, often breeds contempt.

If we are not careful, we can become increasingly enmeshed and the relationship loses its vitality as its original purpose becomes compromised. This is a classic example of *saṃyoga,* where a relationship becomes confused and there is a loss of freedom. *Asteya* and *brahmacarya* become increasingly relevant as an antidote to the potential for this *saṃyoga.*

Asteya is literally 'non-stealing'. This has an obvious meaning in not stealing physical objects. But we must also consider the many ways we can take from another person what is rightly theirs: how we might steal their attention, their ideas, and even profit unfairly from their company and association.

Asteya may be understood as 'not taking advantage of the other'. It is a development of *ahiṃsā* and particularly comes to bear as a relationship deepens. Like *ahiṃsā*, it is concerned with the quality of the space that we offer the other person in a relationship, a space in which they are not exploited or used in any way. According to the Yoga Sūtra, if we can really embrace *asteya* we will receive 'treasures'. The metaphor of treasure, or precious gems (*ratna*), is commonly used in Indian philosophy to indicate the richness of life. So, in fact, through embracing *asteya* we have the possibility of receiving so much more – something that touches life itself, rich and fresh: the product of open and free interaction rather than of grasping and manipulation.

YS 2.38 brahmacarya-pratiṣṭhāyāṃ vīrya-lābhaḥ

For one who maintains priorities, tremendous energy develops

As the twin of *asteya*, *brahmacarya* is concerned with how we maintain our focus in the relationship as it develops. We understand *brahmacarya* as 'not losing our priorities' in the relationship. Literally translated, *brahmacarya* means travelling towards *brahma*, the highest truth, reality or God.

In a traditional context, *brahmacarya* was a stage of life where young people studied the highest truths intensively with a teacher before they married and began family life. For monastic orders, the stage of *brahmacarya* was maintained throughout life. The focus in *brahmacarya* is realising the highest truth, and thus avoiding any distractions or loss of vitality. The most powerful distraction and loss of vitality was considered to arise through sexual activity and hence *brahmacarya* became associated with sexual restraint and often celibacy. The spirit of *brahmacarya* is literally about moving towards the highest truth or, in a more general context, maintaining boundaries so that one does not lose sight of one's goal.

'The focus in brahmacarya is realising the highest truth, and thus avoiding any distractions or loss of vitality.'

Over time, it is easy to find oneself drawn into aspects of a relationship that were not anticipated which can easily become distractions. Sometimes, they may be welcome and appropriate, but often they divert our focus and dissipate our energy.

In a similar way to *asteya*, failure to respect *brahmacarya* can lead to the space and clarity of the relationship becoming compromised. Particularly in professional relationships, such as with work colleagues or in teaching or therapeutic roles, the blurring of boundaries can have serious consequences.

Even for someone established in the other *yama*, they may find themselves manipulated, tempted or coerced into territory that is inappropriate or undesirable in a relationship. In such circumstances, restraint and discipline is needed to maintain appropriate boundaries. For the yoga teacher, Desikachar had some straightforward advice: "When teaching yoga, stick to yoga".[3]

3. Personal communication.

In any situation where we begin to become overwhelmed or consumed beyond what is appropriate, (for example, becoming obsessed with our work), we could say that there is an issue with *brahmacarya*. The fruit of being established in *brahmacarya* is vitality and vigour. *Brahmacarya* helps us to channel our energy and prevents us from dissipating it unwisely. Whenever we feel low in energy, it would be advisable to consider *brahmacarya*, asking ourselves what are our priorities, what is dissipating our energy, and what boundaries need to be put in place or strengthened to protect ourselves.

Even in the West where attitudes towards sexuality may be very different from the traditional Indian context, we would still be wise to recognise the power of our sexual energy and the ways in which it may support us or be abused. This has been the downfall of many spiritual teachers.

Dancing with life: *aparigraha*

YS 2.39 aparigraha-sthairye janma-kathaṃtā-saṃbodhaḥ

When non-grasping is established, the mysteries of life are revealed

Aparigraha means 'non-grasping' or 'non-possession'. At first glance, this might seem synonymous with non-stealing, but the scope of each is quite different. *Aparigraha* concerns the ability to keep a relationship fresh and uncluttered in a much more general sense. It recognises our tendency to allow a relationship to accumulate baggage over time, so that it becomes increasingly defined by what has come before. This is a natural tendency in all relationships, but it fundamentally limits our vitality and freedom. *Aparigraha* is the ultimate antidote for *saṃyoga* in relationships. As the last of the *yama*, it occupies a special place and has a profound significance.

Practising *aparigraha* involves meeting a relationship consistently as if for the first time, letting go of expectations, prejudices and habitual patterns accumulated from the past. In the words of Peter Hersnack, "don't make your relationship into a photo album",[4] where memories invite constant expectation, comparison and disappointment.

'Non grasping' involves letting go of what has been and living in the present. *Aparigraha* is related to *vairāgya*, and like *vairāgya*, can be misunderstood in a way that limits, rather than opens us. Letting go and detaching can easily become an avoidance technique. We are detached, so nothing touches us; we don't hold on to anything, so we don't really care about anything and nothing really matters. Genuine *aparigraha* is none of these. We are present and open to the possibilities of the moment, in a way that allows us to feel and experience fully, but with sensitivity and respect for the other *yama* out of which it arises. It allows us to experience the full richness of life.

The fruit of *aparigraha* is one of the more curious claims of the Yoga Sūtra: by becoming established in *aparigraha* there is an awakening to the 'how-ness of life' (*janma-kathaṃtā*).[5] This suggests that embodying *aparigraha* brings insight into the nature of life itself. This is universal and transcends any specific relationship. It opens our eyes to a universal truth that touches something of the mystery of life. The key to understanding this is to return to the fundamental principles of the yoga worldview – the relationship between spirit and matter: a mysterious relationship that gives rise to life and vitality within us (*prāṇa*). When we live this relationship creatively, we are energised: engaged in life, but also in some sense always free. When we misidentify with this energy of life, crystallising our hopes, fears, and sense of identity in an unhealthy way, we can become increasingly stuck. We also lose the ability to respond creatively to the changes and challenges that life presents.

4. Personal communication.

5. *Katham* is literally 'how' and the suffix *tā* makes a qualitative noun out of the word: hence literally 'how-ness.'

Yama as the 'prāṇāyāma of relationships'

An important principle in yoga is the cultivation of the free flow of *prāṇa*, vital energy. *Prāṇa* flows within the body governing all physiology and psychological processes, but also circulates outside the body in our perception and interaction with the world around us. As we have seen, in Haṭha Yoga, prāṇāyāma is understood as a process by which blockages and restrictions in the body can be removed from the system of energetic channels called *nāḍī*. The free circulation of *prāṇa* brings vitality, clear perception and stability of mind. Blockages in the system create illness, psychological issues and ignorance. Clearing the central channel by removing the fundamental blockage at its base, allowing *prāṇa* to flow where normally it does not, is associated with profound wisdom and deep absorption.[6]

Relationships are also channels through which there is energetic interaction – and *yama* can be understood as the 'prāṇāyāma of relationships'. Often, we create blockages which accumulate over time. The energy in such relationships becomes increasingly stuck and stagnant, and these relationships become subject to projection, manipulation and distortion. The *yama*, like prāṇāyāma, help to free up the energetic channels and to keep them clear, so that the energy of a relationship (which is also seen as *prāṇa*) can circulate freely, remaining vibrant and alive. Mastering *aparigraha* is like clearing the central channel in that it unlocks a far wider scope of experience and vitality.

In prāṇāyāma, unblocking the central *nāḍī* requires considerable preparation; in a similar way, *aparigraha* arises as the fruit of the other *yama*. As the final *yama, aparigraha* allows us to establish freedom in all our relationships and for these relationships to remain vital and fresh as they develop. It is like the 'magic key' that unlocks our experience of life. We should never forget that *aparigraha*, along with the other *yama*, is something that must be practised. Understanding

6. In Krishnamacharya's teachings, the primary blockage which stops *prāṇa* from flowing in the central channel is *kuṇḍalinī*, which he equated with *avidyā*. Thus, one goal of practice is to 'wake up' *kuṇḍalinī/avidyā* so that *prāṇa* can flow unimpeded.

the *yama* can help, but only in as much as they inform our practice, a practice that must extend way beyond the confines of the mat to touch all areas of our lives, and help us to live more creatively and vibrantly.

Sādhana: Countering negative tendencies

YS 2.31 jāti-deśa-kāla-samaya-anavacchinnāḥ sārva-bhaumāḥ mahā-vratam

When yama are observed in all circumstances, irrespective of birth, place or time, it is like a Great Vow

Cultivating *yama*, and perhaps more importantly, addressing the negative tendencies that run counter to them, is a big challenge. In his commentary, Vyāsa acknowledges that under normal circumstances, observance of *yama* is conditional upon our livelihood and culture. A fisherman, for example, cannot observe *ahiṃsā* towards the fish that he catches and kills. Similarly, there are extreme situations that call for responses that contravene the *yama*.

However, if the *yama* are observed in all conditions irrespective of our livelihood, culture or situation, this is considered a *mahāvratam*: a great vow, and a serious undertaking. This is a pathway only for the serious yogi; for most of us, however, it remains an ideal which can inspire us within the realities of our lives.

We should remember that in yoga and Indian philosophy in general, guidelines for conduct such as the *yama* are not simply about being good and morally superior. Nor are *yama* a selfish undertaking – they encourage relationships that are positive for all involved. It is also important to emphasise that *yama* are not imposed for their own sake, but because they are helpful in maintaining our clarity and peace of mind. They are designed to keep matters straightforward, reflecting the truth of how things are and to eliminate negative consequences of our thoughts and actions. The enlightened being does not have to practise *yama*: it is how they naturally are. For us mere mortals, however, very much on the path of practice, *yama* and the reduction of their opposite tendencies is something that we need to actively cultivate. But, as 'trainees', we should have compassion towards ourselves and others when we struggle or fail.

YS 2.33 vitarka-bādhane pratipakṣa-bhāvanam

When we are trapped by (disturbing) thoughts, we can cultivate a different perspective

The Yoga Sūtra suggests a fundamental approach to working with thoughts that run counter to the *yama*, particularly when we feel stuck with such thoughts. The first stage is to recognise them, but even then, it is not always easy to stop them. It is as if they have their own energy, and reinforce each other, even if we want them to stop. This is the sense in which we can feel oppressed or trapped by our negative thoughts and feelings.

In such cases, we work with *pratipakṣa bhāvana*, literally: 'cultivating the other wing'. We find a way to see things differently by deliberately cultivating thoughts or feelings opposite to those that are troubling us. It can also be helpful to remind ourselves of the consequences of negative thoughts and behaviour. At the heart of the method lies a simple truth: we are creatures of habit, even in our emotional and psychological lives. We tend to live through repeated patterns of thought, feeling and behaviour. By deliberately cultivating a different feeling, we are both undermining the existing habit and seeking to create a stronger positive one.

Thus, when we experience thoughts and feelings that run counter to the *yama*, we should cultivate alternatives which are more helpful. There are many ways that we can practise *pratipakṣa bhāvana*; for example, we might formally sit in meditation and imagine a problematic relationship. Then we may consciously generate positive feelings towards the other person that are consistent with the spirit of *yama*.

Another way to understand *pratipakṣa bhāvana* is to change our point of view. We might imagine relating to the other person from a neutral perspective, outside of the relationship. Or, we might imagine the situation from their point of view, as if we were walking in their shoes. These both take us out of our habitual orbits and enable a fresh perspective.

We might also differentiate between the facts of a situation and our story about it. The story is our own construction, and thus it is possible to change it: we could make a conscious effort to 'reframe our story'. By understanding a situation in a new way, a new space for perception is cleared.

YS 2.34 vitarkāḥ hiṃsā-ādayaḥ kṛta-kārita-anumoditāḥ lobha-krodha-moha-pūrvakāḥ mṛdu-madhya-adhimātrāḥ duḥkha-ajñāna ananta-phalāḥ iti pratipakṣa-bhāvanam

Disturbing thoughts, arising from desire, anger or delusion, whether acted upon or tacit, and of whatever intensity, will result in endless suffering and confusion. So: cultivate alternative perspectives

The Yoga Sūtra emphasises the negative effects that accumulate when we indulge emotions that run contrary to *yama*. These are said to be *duḥkha*, personal suffering and a sense of dissatisfaction, and *ajñāna*, misunderstanding and confusion. It is in our own interests to practise the *yama* as a means to reduce distress and suffering in our relationships, and to live with greater clarity. Patañjali also identifies the root negative emotions that violate the *yama*: *lobha* (desire), *krodha* (anger), and *moha* (delusion). When these predominate, our actions cause distress and misunderstanding. By taking small steps to live in accordance with the *yama*, we work towards reducing such negative consequences. The more we can embrace the *yama*, the freer we become. No effort is wasted.

Chapter 12

शौचसंतोषतपःस्वाध्यायेश्वरप्रणिधानानि
नियमाः ।

Living with Ourselves

YS 2.32 śauca-saṃtoṣa-tapaḥ-svādhyāya-īśvara-praṇidhānāni niyamāḥ

The niyama are self-care, contentment, purifying discipline, self-enquiry and a trust in the process of Life

The *niyama* are the second of the eight limbs of *aṣṭāṅga yoga*. They are five attitudes, or restraints, presented by Patañjali to free us from unhelpful habits and thereby guide us to greater independence and peace of mind. Like the *yama*, they can be structured as an initial pair (setting the basic conditions), a subsequent pair (providing the means to go deeper), and a final *niyama* that takes us beyond ourselves to far greater horizons.

They are given as a list in YS 2.32 and then an additional sūtra is offered for each *niyama* that describes the results when it is mastered and applied. This structure mirrors the sūtras on *yama*.

The first of the *niyama, śauca,* is self-care, often translated as 'cleanliness'. Heading the list, it has a special place – the others are the means to refine and condition it. Although 'cleanliness' may appear to be relatively superficial, it assumes a new significance when understood as the profound cultivation of lightness and clarity (*sattva guṇa*) in body and mind. It is both a starting point and an important goal: *sattva* is the support within our minds for the most profound realisation. Patañjali distinguishes inner *śauca* (psychological) from outer *śauca* (bodily), and two sūtras, YS 2.40 and 2.41, give the fruits of each. *Śauca*, often quickly glossed over, is fundamental and central to the yoga path.

The second *niyama, saṃtoṣa,* is 'contentment' and shifts the emphasis from the material (i.e. our body and mind) towards the spiritual. Here, freedom from desire and transcending the duality of 'normal' happiness and unhappiness, is the path to a deeper contentment. *Saṃtoṣa* is the means to be profoundly at ease within ourselves.

The three remaining *niyama* are the components of *kriyā yoga* and we shall discuss these further in Chapter 13. Through *tapas* (discipline) and *svādhyāya* (study, listening), we refine our relationship with ourselves to actively deepen our *śauca* and *saṃtoṣa. Tapas* is more concerned with working on the material (including the mind), while *svādhyāya* takes us more inward towards the spiritual Self. *Īśvara praṇidhāna,* the last *niyama,* has a similar position to *aparigraha* in the framework of the *yama. Īśvara praṇidhāna*, a trust in the process of Life, requires that we consider our relationship to forces beyond our control and our place within the greater world order. We explore this in Chapter 16.

The basis of a healthy relationship with ourselves

We can explore *niyama* using a similar framework to the *yama*: as two pairs plus one. Whereas two *yama* focus on the other person in a relationship, and two focus on oneself, with the *niyama,* two concern the outer aspects of our being and two the inner.

	Outer aspects of our being	Inner aspects of our being
Establishing the basis for independence from unhelpful habits	*śauca* Self-care and cleanliness	*saṃtoṣa* Contentment
The means to deepen the practice	*tapas* Discipline	*svādhyāya* Self-enquiry
Going beyond ourselves	*īśvara praṇidhāna* Trust in the process of Life	

Śauca is about how we care for ourselves and our environment, and is thus more outer. *Saṃtoṣa* is more inner, concerned with a contentment arising from our very being. Thus, the focus of *śauca* is the material *(prakṛti)*, while *saṃtoṣa's* focus is linked more to the spiritual *(puruṣa)*. *Śauca* and *saṃtoṣa* are the basis of a healthy relationship with ourselves: we are content and at ease, we care for ourselves and we live in a way that supports lightness and clarity.

Śauca and *saṃtoṣa* are a profound and important part of the practice and, as with so many of the principles of the Yoga Sūtra, they have multiple levels. Whilst these first two establish the foundations of the *niyama*, it is also important to consider our motivations in practising yoga. There are likely to be many factors that draw us to the teachings and the practice. The *Haṭha Yoga Pradīpikā* warns of *graha niyama*,[1] which Krishnamacharya understood as a self-discipline that is maintained too tightly, or for the wrong reasons. For many yoga practitioners, aspects of the

1. HYP 1.15

practice can reinforce or indulge unhealthy motivations. Is our preoccupation with āsana largely driven by a desire to cultivate the body or stay slim? Does *puruṣa* offer a promise of life beyond death and salve our basic existential fears? Are we adopting a philosophy that allows us to reject a society and culture that we simply cannot cope with? Perhaps this is inevitable to a degree, but we should be clear about why we are drawn to some things and not others. Often what really drives us is not immediately apparent, and it is important to be vigilant. The principle of *ahiṃsā* applies to ourselves as well as to others, and we must be careful that we do not simply reinforce our own subtle psychological pathologies, or engage in a pursuit that verges on self-abuse. *Niyama* held 'too tightly' could be just that. *Niyama* – and *śauca/saṃtoṣa* in particular – should help to establish a healthy relationship with ourselves.

Śauca: Cultivating lightness and clarity

YS 2.40 śaucāt svāṅga-jugupsā parair asaṃsargaḥ

From self-care arises a lack of obsession with our own bodies, and a reduction of infatuation with those of others

Peter Hersnack interpreted *śauca* as "caring for oneself as if for another".[2] It is often translated as 'purity', but this can feel too austere – such as wearing a hair shirt in order to purify our sins. Alternatively, as stated above, it may be translated as 'cleanliness' – but this feels too superficial. *Śauca* as 'self-care', however, has a more nurturing feel to it: it invites us to look after ourselves in a way which is tender and protective. Often it is easier to take care of someone else – a loved one, a relative or even a pet. We may trivialise our own needs in a way that we would not if we were caring for another. Mistaken ideas about yoga, detachment from the world and the rejection of material things can reinforce such tendencies. For some, neglecting cleanliness, appearance

2. Personal communication.

and other elements of self-care can indicate (misplaced) spiritual superiority. But 'caring for oneself as if for another' asks us to value ourselves and consider how our bodies and minds can be a fit support for an experience of yoga. However, 'caring for ourselves' can also easily become confused with self-indulgence or neurotic concerns about our health.

The Sanskrit root of *śauca* is 'to shine' or 'gleam', which are both associated with *sattva guṇa*. *Sattva guṇa* has the qualities of lightness and clarity, and as we have seen, the Sanskrit for clarity is *prakāśa* – 'that which shines'. Thus, *śauca* is fundamentally linked to the cultivation of *sattva*. In popular culture, caring for oneself and treating oneself kindly can easily be equated with sensual indulgence. In deciding what really qualifies as *śauca* the acid test should be: does it cultivate *sattva* in our bodies and minds? Does it encourage a feeling of physical, emotional and mental lightness and clarity? We are not against chocolate brownies (in moderation!), but honestly: do they encourage *sattva*? *Śauca* requires a degree of discrimination and often, self-discipline.

Peter Hersnack told a memorable story concerning *śauca*.[3] There were two children in a family, one of whom was seriously ill. The family rallied around the sick child, who became the focus of the parents' attention, and the centre of family life. As this situation continued, the child who was well became more withdrawn and alienated, almost invisible. In the last hundred years or so, yoga has become increasingly associated with maintaining one's health and youthfulness, and yoga therapy has become popular for addressing many physical or mental conditions. It is certainly true that yoga and āyurveda share many common principles, and yoga may be a very effective therapeutic tool, but it is important to not lose sight of the goal. For yoga to truly address the fundamental causes of human suffering we must explore the deeper nature of ourselves and that potential. *Śauca* needs to care for our

3. Association of Yoga Studies Convention, Shropshire, UK July 2012.

'sick child' but also, and perhaps most importantly, care and nurture our 'well child'. We must be careful we do not become so fixated on our niggles and problems that we lose sight of our possibilities and potentials. 'Caring for ourselves as if for another' importantly includes caring for *the part of us that is not problematic*. As we age and physical challenges arise, it is easy to become preoccupied with, and increasingly defined by, one's problems. *Śauca* takes us beyond this.

Śauca is unusual among the *yama* and *niyama* in that it has two sūtras discussing its fruits. The first (YS 2.40) discusses outer *śauca*, concerned principally with the body. This difficult sūtra can easily be misinterpreted. Two results are given, *svāṅga jugupsā* and *parair asaṃsargaḥ*. The first is usually translated as a 'distaste' or 'disgust' for the body (*svāṅga* means 'one's own limbs'). There was certainly a current in Indian thought at the time of the Yoga Sūtra that viewed the body in a negative light, as something to be defeated, an obstacle to spiritual pursuits. However, we consider this to be unhelpful. It is true that attending to the needs of the body takes considerable time and energy, and ultimately, the body is subject to decay. In this sense, we could say that we become aware of the limitations of the body and whilst attending to it, we should not become overly preoccupied or attached to it.

The root of the word *jugupsā*, is *gup*, meaning 'to protect' or 'keep secret'. We can understand *śauca* of the body as a means to protect the body, to look after it and, on a deeper level, to protect us *from* the body by minimising the distraction that it causes (because it is functioning as well as possible). A deeper understanding still, suggests that by realising the limitations and frailties of the body, we do not get caught up in it. Krishnamacharya was quoted as saying "what use is the sword of knowledge if the bearer is too weak to wield it?"[4] Although the mind can transcend the body's pain, it is not easy to maintain our clarity when there is a lot of physical discomfort. As we have seen, in Chapter 4, the

4. We have heard this story from both Desikachar and from Paul Harvey.

sūtra *heyaṃ duḥkham anāgataṃ* (YS 2.16) encourages us to avoid the pain and distress that can be avoided and outer *śauca* has an important role in this.

The other fruit of outer *śauca*, *parair asaṃsarga*, means 'lack of contact with others' and it addresses the effect of others and our environment upon us. *Śauca* here encourages us to favour *satsaṅga* – association that is supportive and consistent with our goals. Although there have been yogis who have lived and practised anonymously in the most challenging conditions, often yogis have favoured solitude or living within communities of like-minded souls. We are prone to be influenced by others and absorb their qualities. Whilst life often requires us to engage in difficult situations (much compassionate activity involves working with difficult people or challenging situations and environments), it is not easy to maintain one's balance in such situations and we should be mindful of the toll it takes. Part of the practise of *śauca* is to cleanse oneself of the negative effects of such circumstances, and also to explore choices that reduce or eliminate situations or relationships that are unnecessarily toxic.

In his commentary concerning outer *śauca*, Vyāsa gives some examples, such as discipline about food and the performance of rituals of purification. For Krishnamacharya and Desikachar too, diet was very important because it influences both our body and our state of mind. The inclusion of ritual is also interesting here. Because ritual purity is such an important concern of traditional Brahmanical society, it would be easy to dismiss this aspect of *śauca* as culturally specific. But in the modern therapy world, the need for supervision to help unburden the therapist from the negative influences of clients and their stories is well acknowledged. Perhaps many of us have the need for some kind of purification from difficult situations in our lives.

YS 2.41 sattva-śuddhi saumanasya ekāgrya indriyajaya ātma-darśana-yogyatvāni ca

And (the development) of a clear mind, positive attitude, focus, control of the senses and a fitness for a deep experience of the Self

This sūtra presents five fruits of inner *śauca*:

1 *sattva-śuddhi* – a clear mind
2 *saumanasya* – positive attitude
3 *ekāgrya* – focus
4 *indriya-jaya* – control of the senses
5 *ātma-darśana-yogyatva* – fitness for a deep experience of the Self

As with many of the other lists in the Yoga Sūtra, the first can be seen as the foundation and most important, and the last also has a special significance. The first, *sattva-śuddhi,* suggests that through *śauca* we can promote *sattva* in our minds. This emphasises the essential qualification for *śauca*: that it cultivates and inclines us towards *sattva*. And in a similar way to *ahiṃsā* in relation to the other *yama*, we can see the other fruits of inner *śauca* as arising from, and in some sense qualifying and enhancing, *sattva śuddhi.*

The second fruit is *saumanasya*, a cheerful or positive attitude. The opposite, *daurmanasya* (literally 'bad mind'), is negative or pessimistic thinking. *Daurmanasya* always involves excessive *tamas*, which contributes to a distorted view, and then further *tamas* which contributes to a heavy or depressed state. *Rajas*, leading to anxiety, neurotic or obsessive thinking, may also be out of balance. *Saumanasya* requires the light, clear and spacious qualities of *sattva* which give rise to clarity of thinking.

One-pointedness (*ekāgrya*) is the third fruit. This is a natural consequence of the reduction of *rajas* and *tamas* and the cultivation of *sattva*. *Ekāgrya* is the level of *citta vṛtti nirodha* that we can actively practise and cultivate. The necessity for *sattva* in order to direct the mind with clarity and stability is emphasised throughout the text and equated with the highest states of yoga. In this sense, all effective yoga practice **is** *śauca*: the cultivation of *sattva*.

The Sanskrit term for the senses is *indriya*.[5] A recurrent theme in the Indian spiritual tradition is how the senses can easily become the masters, keeping us enslaved to the sensations they provide. This is the opposite to their ideal role as servants of the Self. For the senses to bind us, *rajas* and *tamas* must be dominant in the mind. *Rajas* stimulates the desire for sensual pleasure and *tamas* deludes us into believing that the *indriya* are masters, not servants. *Sattva* is the antidote to this situation, providing the clarity to understand the true nature of the *indriya* and to use them wisely. Thus, the fourth of the fruits of *śauca* is *indriya jaya*: mastery of the senses. Here, we use the senses with clarity and skill – to nurture, rather than imprison us.

The last of the fruits of *śauca*, like the last of the *yama*, takes us beyond the immediate concerns of the others. It is *ātma darśana yogyatva*: making us fit for a vision of the true self. The domain of *śauca* is *prakṛti*, that which is subject to the *guṇa* and therefore can be purified. The Self, *ātma*, cannot be purified because it is beyond the *guṇa*. Here what is suggested is a vision or realisation of the Self – and this experience *can only happen in the mind*. Ironically, the mind itself is the means to realise the truth *beyond* the mind. We work with the mind to transcend it (or at least to realise its true nature and role: as a servant of its lord). What are the conditions in the mind that make such a realisation possible? The answer, of course, is a prevalence of *sattva guṇa*; we might say that *sattva* is the support for the experience of *puruṣa* or *ātma*. This final aspect of *śauca* elevates it to a principle of the highest importance as it is an essential support for the deepest of experiences. Although this might sound rather abstract, in fact it has great practical relevance. Even the relative cultivation of *sattva* (moving from a position of less *sattva* to more *sattva*) creates the conditions for deeper experiences and realisations. The principal is quite universal.

5. *Indriya* are discussed in considerable detail in Chapter 14.

Being content with what is

YS 2.42 saṃtoṣād anuttamaḥ sukha-lābhaḥ

From contentment arises a happiness which is unexcelled

Saṃtoṣa means 'contentment', and in particular a contentment that comes from within. It is linked inwards to the spiritual aspect of ourselves (as distinct from *śauca,* which is more concerned with *prakṛti*). Developing *saṃtoṣa* gives rise to *sukha anuttamaḥ,* a happiness that is unexcelled. This is beyond normal *sukha,* which has an opposite, *duḥkha.* It is beyond all qualities such as pleasure and suffering, or happiness that arises from external conditions. When discussing the *kleśa* we met *rāga* (desire) and *dveṣa* (aversion). These result in a temporary, ordinary level of happiness when a desire is fulfilled or something successfully avoided, or an experience of *duḥkha* when they are not. But *kleśa,* by definition, ultimately give rise to suffering. Thus any satisfaction arising from *kleśa* is short-lived and unsatisfactory. The *sukha* arising from *saṃtoṣa* is of a completely different order and hence the qualification that it is unsurpassed: *anuttamaḥ.*

So, what could be the source of such *sukha*? The answer is realisation of *puruṣa.* In the Upaniṣads,[6] the nature of the Self is said to be *satcitānanda* – real, conscious and blissful. Elsewhere, including in the Yoga Sūtra, we understand that the Self is beyond qualities (*nirguṇa*). This gives us an apparent contradiction until we realise that although the Self is beyond qualities, an experience of it must arise within the mind, which is subject to the *guṇa.* Thus *saṃtoṣa* becomes possible as our link to what is inside becomes stronger. The support for such a realisation is *sattva,* the result of *śauca.* Hence *śauca* here also functions as a foundation for *saṃtoṣa.*

As embodied beings, our minds and the world we live in are subject to all three *guṇa.* Diligently cultivating *sattva* will not necessarily stop the domination of the other *guṇa* at times. But if we trust our connection to our deepest Being,

6. Ancient Vedic texts predating the Yoga Sūtra which describe the mystical experiences of Self-realisation.

beyond the *guṇa*, a special type of contentment arises. According to yoga, *prāṇa* is the manifestation of *puruṣa*, or Life within us; *prāṇa* is to Life what sunlight is to the sun. We experience *prāṇa* as a feeling of being alive, even when we are in pain, despair or depression. *Prāṇa* is thus the sign that *puruṣa* is present. As a practical definition, we could understand *saṃtoṣa* as a contentment that arises from feeling that one is carried by Life from inside, irrespective of what is happening, or how we are feeling from moment to moment. Cultivating *sattva* is certainly a means to developing our understanding and strengthening our connection to the deeper parts of ourselves. But real *saṃtoṣa* is tested by our experience of life in all its forms. *Sukha anuttamaḥ* gives us an ability to be with what is, *whatever* its form or qualities; it is not simply the bliss of deep meditation or idyllic circumstances.

It is natural to want to make the best of our lives. Too often, however, this becomes an obsession – an endless search for the perfect relationship, perfect clothes, perfect social life, perfect family, etc. *Saṃtoṣa* is accepting that we have a good enough life. This is not an invitation to be complacent or without aspiration, but to take the pressure off expectation. Life is a gift which arises from inside, whatever form it may take, and there is profound contentment that can come from truly allowing it to be our fundamental support and refuge, whether in tears or laughter, joy or despair. Life is our common denominator, for as long as we have the privilege of being alive.

The principles of *viniyoga* and *vinyāsa krama* invite us to start where we are and progress in steps. Strategies to develop contentment at a practical level can be very useful. Cultivating gratitude in our lives and noticing the richness and delightfulness in many simple things, such as nature, can be a powerful antidote to everyday dissatisfaction. Taking more time over small things, and cultivating simplicity in life, can give us space to appreciate what we have. We may discover that we already have much more *sukha* available to us in our lives than we ever thought possible. However, we should not confuse this with *sukha anuttamaḥ*, which arises from inside and is independent of our success or failure, sickness or health, flexibility or stiffness.

Saṃtoṣa is not simply the *appearance* of benevolent beatitude – a common mask in yoga circles. *Saṃtoṣa* is linked to *satya* (truth) – it requires authenticity and is based on both the reality of where life comes from, and the reality of the *form* that life is taking (i.e. what is happening), without illusions and free of any expectation that it should be different.

Like *vairāgya*, *saṃtoṣa* can be misunderstood as a kind of armour that protects us from the world. We might think that contentment is only possible if we withdraw and remain disengaged. Here we cannot be threatened, as if we are living in an ivory tower. But this may well be a fragile state, and also a tragic one if we value the process and richness of life. True *saṃtoṣa* gives us the contentment to be in life while connected to something beyond it. It gives us the freedom and joy to be really touched by life and death without being destroyed by either. This does not mean that we should not make choices about how we live and what we expose ourselves to – life need not be an endurance test! But importantly, *saṃtoṣa* (indeed, yoga as a whole) should not become an excuse to hide from life.

Sādhana: Looking after ourselves

Taking care in our practice

The scope of yoga, and *yama* and *niyama* in particular, is broad, covering every aspect of our lives. In very physically oriented approaches there can be a tendency to apply the eight limbs, including *yama* and *niyama*, exclusively to the physical sphere, presenting yoga as a purely mat-based practice system. This distorts and reduces yoga to a fraction of its intended scope. With this said, however, we can apply the principles of *yama* and *niyama* to our physical practice just as we can to all other aspects of our lives, and here we would like to discuss 'taking care' in our practice.

Over its long and varied history, the yoga tradition has explored all manner of physical and meditative practices, which in some cases have pushed the physical limits of the body to the extreme. A common Haṭha Yoga practice, for example, involved cutting the fraenum of the tongue allowing it to be unnaturally extended and turned back in the mouth in a practice known as *khecarī*. Krishnamacharya was strongly against such practices: in accordance with the fundamental principle of *ahiṃsā*, he believed yoga practice should not harm the body and certainly should not include its deliberate mutilation. Indeed, he was against all practices that introduced foreign substances into the body, even with the purpose of purification, believing that air and fire (in the sense of breath and the 'internal fire', *agni*) were sufficient to cleanse the system.[7]

We have defined *śauca* as 'taking care of ourselves as if of another' and linked *śauca* to the cultivation of *sattva*. So the question is how to ensure that our practice both does us no harm on the one hand, and on the other, supports us in taking care of ourselves. As ever, we must bear in mind the process of *pariṇāma* (change) that inevitably bears upon our bodies as we mature and age. The *sat viniyoga* (wholesome application) of yoga must ensure that the practice remains both supportive of us and certainly not injurious to our wellbeing.

Being kind to ourselves, and the dangers of projection

As with most alternative health practitioners, yoga teachers will sometimes hear their students express surprise (and often disappointment) if they become ill.

7. Krishnamacharya did not accept the practices listed in texts such as the *Haṭha Yoga Pradīpikā* which used cloth or water to cleanse the body of excess *kapha*. He believed these were corrupted practices from āyurveda that were often inappropriately used.

"You shouldn't have a cold – you're a yoga teacher!" they might say. These projections can take other forms too: "do you ever get stressed?" or "are you ever angry?". It's worth realising that one of the reasons that many of us took up yoga is because there was something fundamental in our lives that we felt needed addressing – yoga is there to help us deal with our 'issues'!

While it is true that yoga practice done well and appropriately optimises good health, both physical and mental, we will all have our ups and downs. This is only natural. It is also true that sometimes illness can be unexpected and perplexing; it seemed unbelievable that Desikachar, a truly focused and inspiring teacher and practitioner of yoga, should start suffering from dementia at a comparatively early age.[8] Similarly, Peter Hersnack died very quickly from an aggressive form of cancer in 2016 in his late sixties. Yoga is not a universal inoculation from illness or death; it can, however, help us to deal with them as they arise.

It is easy to become disillusioned or disappointed if we fall ill or find life a struggle, and we can make our conditions even worse if we feel guilty or unworthy as well. If *śauca* is 'to treat ourselves as we would another', it is important that we extend compassion to ourselves when we need to, and acknowledge our vulnerabilities, imperfections and weaknesses. This is not the same as indulging them – it is treating ourselves with care.

A practice for cultivating *saṃtoṣa*

Evolutionary psychologists have frequently pointed out that we are hard-wired to look for danger and consequently we can be hypervigilant towards anything untoward. Dangers are a threat, and they need to be noticed. We also perceive faults far more acutely than we do successes – a single word of criticism can sting amongst a sea of praise. When things are going well we often take them for

8. It is not clear when his condition started, but by his seventies Desikachar was quite ill and sadly passed away in 2016 at the age of 78.

granted and do not notice them. As the old soul song says: "You don't miss your water till your well runs dry!" It is all too easy to develop amnesia for all the positives in our lives, whilst maintaining and harbouring grudges for far too long. We forget what we should remember, and remember what we should forget. Because this is in some ways natural, we need to work at cultivating its opposite – to noticing the good and to take in what will nourish us, rather than what will eventually poison us.

We have found a simple practice, done at the end of āsana or prāṇāyāma, to be extremely effective.[9] We sit down and let the breath and thoughts relax. Then, as we slowly breathe in, we allow somebody – anybody – to enter into our minds. As we then exhale, we offer them thanks – for whatever. On the next breath, we wait to see who will appear, who we can next offer thanks to. It may be the same person, and of course certain people in our lives may appear more regularly than others. But what is most interesting is that completely surprising people appear – friends or acquaintances we have not thought about for years. The boy who sat next to you in school when you were five, or a stranger you smiled at on a bus. It doesn't have to be profound, it is simply a gesture of connection and gratitude and it works. On many occasions Ranju has smiled as he practises this, remembering and being with certain people in his life – even for just a breath. It is a simple and accessible practice that helps us cultivate a profound sense of connection and contentment – and it need take as few as twelve breaths or so.

9. This beautiful practice has elements of prāṇāyāma and also links to the Buddhist meditation practice of *metta bhāvana*. It was taught to us in 2015 in a workshop with our friend Navtej Johar, another student of T.K.V. Desikachar.

Chapter 13

तपः स्वाध्यायेश्वरप्रणिधानानि
क्रियायोगः ।

Working on Ourselves

YS 2.1 tapaḥ-svādhyāya-īśvara-praṇidhānāni kriyā-yogaḥ

The yoga of action consists of observing certain disciplines, reflecting on the nature of oneself and trusting in the process of life

Tapas, svādhyāya and *īśvara praṇidhāna,* the last three members of the *niyama,* are also presented independently at the beginning of the second chapter of the Yoga Sūtra as the components of *kriyā yoga,* the yoga of action. Here they stand alone and begin the chapter on *sādhana. Tapas* (discipline) and *svādhyāya* (self-reflection) are such important principles in the yoga tradition that we are giving them their own chapter here and we shall then discuss *īśvara praṇidhāna* (trusting in the process of life) in more detail in Chapter 16.

Tapas is one of the most ancient and enduring concepts associated with spiritual practice in India. Myths in the Upaniṣads locate *tapas* at the heart of the creative process and there are many stories describing how sages, saints and demons have gained special powers or favours from the gods through *tapas. Tapas* is implied in all serious practices of yoga and it is impossible to understand the transformation process of yoga without some appreciation of *tapas.*

Tapas involves observing certain disciplines which challenge us, and thereby generate 'heat'. This heat is like the fuel of change and transformation, giving us vitality and strength to pursue our goals. Genuine spiritual practice inevitably challenges our habitual patterns of thinking and behaviour, and without some element of *tapas*, our practice lacks 'teeth'. The domain of *tapas* is the material: it is concerned with the transformation of our *prakṛti*, our body and minds, through setting limits on our activity and behaviour. In this way, we can understand *tapas* as engaging with our outer supports.

Svādhyāya invites us to take a journey towards ourselves and to see this also as an important source of transformation and support. Literally translated as 'moving towards our self', it is usually understood as the process of self-enquiry and reflection. The domain of *svādhyāya* is *sva* (Self, or *puruṣa*), and so in this sense the direction of *svādhyāya* is different to *tapas* (whose direction is *prakṛti*). *Svādhyāya* is focused on deepening our understanding and experience of Self, and thus invites us to discover and utilise our inner supports.

Kriyā yoga as a fundamental definition of yoga practice

Although the 'eight limbs' is by far the best-known formulation of yoga practice, *kriyā yoga* as defined in YS 2.1 is more succinct and cuts to the heart of the matter.[1] It is presented at the start of the second chapter of the Yoga Sūtra (entitled *Sādhana Pāda,* the chapter on practice), and is traditionally understood as aimed at the average practitioner grappling to develop a stable mind and struggling with the fears and concerns that afflict us all. *Kriyā yoga,* the yoga of action, tells us what we need to do, or at least the elements that must be included in what we do, to get our practice moving. It is an elaboration of *abhyāsa* and *vairāgya*, our fundamental methodology, and less abstract yet more concise than the eight limbs. As the very first sūtra in the second chapter, we would be foolish to underestimate its importance.

The components of *kriyā yoga* are all important concepts in the Indian tradition in their own right and together create an inclusive model of practice. Certain practices such as chanting, or āsana, might fit more obviously with one of the three 'limbs'. *Tapas, svādhyāya* and *īśvara praṇidhāna* could be seen as different boxes in which to place elements of our practice (with the implication that at some point we should have something in each 'box'). Such a perspective has value, but we should also think of the three elements as being qualities or principles that need to be present to varying degrees in *all* practices. Vedic chanting, for example, when practised diligently and correctly, includes aspects of *tapas, svādhyāya* and *īśvara praṇidhāna*. These are such important ideas that, as teachers, we would be happier if our students were more familiar with the three limbs of *kriyā yoga* than the eight limbs of *aṣṭāṅga*!

1. Some scholars believe *kriyā yoga* was the original formulation and that *aṣṭāṅga yoga* was a later addition to the Yoga Sūtra, perhaps as a reflection of the Buddhist Eight-fold Path. The yoga tradition certainly does not understand things in this way, and sees the complete Yoga Sūtra as a harmonious whole in its current form. In this context *aṣṭāṅga yoga* is seen as a more complete and demanding expression of the practice, whereas *kriyā yoga* is the starting point embodying the essential principles to begin working on ourselves.

Tapas: Purifying ourselves through external means

Tapas is the starting point. The word derives from the root *tap* meaning 'to heat' and it is usually thought of as the cultivation of purifying practices which heat the system and 'burn off the dross' (whether physical or psychological). The commitment to a practice or discipline creates a certain friction and heat. It can (and usually does) include dietary restriction, exercise, regulation of speech and so forth. *Tapas* involves challenging oneself – but not so much as to create a violent reaction. Slow but complete cooking is far preferable than burning one side and leaving the other side raw![2]

Tapas is a fundamental principle in Indian spirituality from ancient times, and appears repeatedly in the Veda, Upaniṣads and later texts. In the *Praśna Upaniṣad*, for example, there is a creation myth where the primordial person (*Prajāpati*, Lord of all creatures), finding himself alone and desiring offspring, creates all living beings through his *tapas*. This illustrates *tapas* as an essential principle not only in practice, but at the very heart of the creative process itself. *Tapas* is essential to our transformation since it is the process of creative change that operates in the evolution of the whole world – the yogi is simply harnessing this fundamental process within themselves.

There are also many stories in which *tapas* is the means to procure special powers and favours from the gods. This is a recurrent theme in the great Indian epic, *The Mahābhārata,* where warriors win special boons from the gods through their extreme discipline. In the story of Bhagīratha, the sage stood on one leg with the heel raised (*bhagīrathāsana*) until Brahma and Śiva responded to his *tapas*, and brought water back to the earth through the goddess Gaṅgā (personifying the river Ganges). When confronted with extreme determination to withstand the rigours of *tapas,* the gods have no option but to respond and

2. Krishnamacharya uses the concept of *paripāka* – 'cooked on all sides' – to describe the gradual elimination of our misunderstanding through the varied and all-inclusive practices of yoga. Other methods might produce rapid results, but are potentially unbalancing if they do not address the whole being.

reward the *tapasvin*, even if they are a demon as in the case of Hiraṇyakaśipu in the story of Narasimha.[3]

In India there has been a long tradition of extreme *tapas* amongst ascetics that has extended the principle to the mortification of the physical body (for example, holding one arm aloft for years). The term *tapas* is frequently translated as 'austerity'. Desikachar was very keen to distance himself from this understanding of *tapas*. *Tapas* should be consistent with the principle of *ahiṃsā* in not harming the body, and supporting *śauca*, the purification and care of ourselves in order to promote *sattva*. This sets certain limits and criteria for the direction of our *tapas*: it is certainly not discipline for discipline's sake, or some perverse and masochistic exercise in self-abuse.

Tapas, in our understanding, involves staying with a discipline or practice in which we are challenged. The boundaries or limits imposed by our *tapas* are really supports that enable us to confront our limitations or habitual patterns, and move beyond them. The ability to take support on dietary restrictions, on āsana, prāṇāyāma and meditative practices, or any other form of discipline, is always there; we needn't wait until tomorrow. They just need to be done! These supports are 'external': the discipline is concerned with something external to us – an activity, pattern of thought, or moderation in food – and therefore in the realm of *prakṛti* and the *guṇa*. Peter Hersnack described *tapas* as "taking external support seriously".[4] Relating to the boundaries of our *tapas* as supports that help us to grow, rather than as restrictions, can lighten the process and inspire us to stay with what otherwise might feel punitive and miserable. In the context of *kriyā yoga*, *tapas* involves a commitment to address one's habits, to begin to challenge oneself, and to move in a new direction. It also generates 'edge' and energy in our lives, which spur us on to greater reflection and prevent us from becoming complacent.

3. The demon Hiraṇyakaśipu was so angry at Viṣṇu for killing his demon brother that he performed *tapas* until Brahma had no option but to respond. He declares that Hiraṇyakaśipu cannot be killed during the day or night, inside or outside, by god, demon, man or animal. Viṣṇu's ingenious response is to take the form of Narasimha, half-man and half-lion, and finally slays the demon at sunset on the threshold of his palace. Narasimha is popular as protector against evil, and a favourite of Krishnamacharya who saw in his leonine body the Haṭha Yoga ideal of broad expanded chest with lower belly drawn in and up, reflecting Krishnamacharya's approach to yogic breathing and the use of *bandha*.

4. Personal communication.

Tapas and *niyama*

YS 2.43 kāya-indriya-siddhiḥ aśuddhi-kṣayāt tapasaḥ

Through discipline comes a mastery of body and senses, and a reduction of impurities

There is a convention that Patañjali adopts in a number of places in the Yoga Sūtra whereby one or more sūtra define the essential nature of something, one or more sūtra explore how to cultivate or deepen it, and one or more sūtra present the fruits. The sūtra on āsana are a good example of this where a single sūtra is used for definition, method and result respectively (YS 2.46–48). Prāṇāyāma, *yama* and indeed *niyama* can also be considered in this way. From this perspective, the essential components of *niyama* are *śauca* and *saṃtoṣa*, and *tapas* is the means to deepen and actively work on *śauca*. This helps to focus our understanding of *tapas*: since *śauca* is inextricably linked to the cultivation of *sattva*, the goal of *tapas* must be the same. In practice, the cultivation of *sattva* is achieved by the reduction of excess *rajas and tamas* and this is the role of *tapas*.

The fruit of *tapas* is given as mastery of body and senses (*kāya-indriya-siddhi*) and a reduction in impurities (*aśuddhi-kṣaya*). Maintaining *tapas* develops self-control, and thus mastery of body and senses. New students often see yoga as a recreational activity to be enjoyed. There is nothing wrong in enjoying your practice, but for *tapas* to be effective there must be an element of challenge and this may mean putting up with a certain discomfort, maybe physical, but most likely psychological.
A.G. Mohan describes *tapas* as "putting up with the discomfort that comes from changing our habits".[5] *Tapas* challenges our habitual patterns and our ability to stay with something even when it no longer glitters, when it becomes boring or uncomfortable. Sometimes in practice, you don't have to like it, you just have to do it!

5. Personal communication.

Traditionally, when you were given a practice by your teacher, that was what you did – nothing more, and nothing less, until you were given a different practice. This did not mean that there was no dialogue, and we should remember that the principles of *ahiṃsā* must always be respected; but essentially staying with the practice was a *tapas*. We do not all have enlightened teachers who we can rely on to give us the right practice, but there is a common tendency for yoga practitioners to 'listen' to their body on a daily basis and do what they 'intuitively need'. Whilst this may be appropriate at times, there is a danger that we will simply do what we feel like doing and thereby undermine the principle of staying with one thing. This is not *tapas*.

Both our bodies and our minds respond to training. Through *tapas* we can develop both mental and physical strength. This requires *abhyāsa*: repeated practice over a long time undertaken with care, enthusiasm and respect. Although *tapas* places constraints upon us, if we relate to them in the right way we can understand *tapas* as 'putting supports in place' to help us grow. *Tapas* is an expression of *abhyāsa*, our fundamental practice principle.

There is a strong training element in yoga, which includes our bodies, our breath and our minds. Responding too easily to sensations in the body or distractions of senses enslaves us to them. Intelligently resisting them, within the boundaries of our *tapas*, brings mastery of body and senses. However, we must be careful that our *tapas* is appropriate and skilfully directed. If we were to reduce yoga to its essential principles, *tapas* would have to be very high up on the list.

The other fruit of *tapas* is *aśuddhi-kṣayāt*, the removal of impurities in the system. This links *tapas* directly to *śauca* as reduction in impurities and the cultivation of *sattva* are two sides of the same coin. These impurities may be physical, energetic or psychological. The emphasis in the Yoga Sūtra is clearly on psychological purification: the removal of habits and conditioning that are unhelpful, lead to suffering, and ultimately distort our perception and understanding. In Haṭha Yoga, the link between the mind and our physiology is emphasised so that an important theme becomes the physical purification of the body and the energetic system through which body and mind are linked. However, even with the emphasis on physical and energetic purification, we should not forget the goal. The *Haṭha Yoga Pradīpikā* repeatedly states that the practices of *haṭha* are only there to serve the goal of *rāja yoga*[6] namely the purification of the mind in order to realise its potential for profound experience and insight in meditation.

This emphasis on purification of the body is also a concern of āyurveda which acknowledges the sum total of all influences upon the human system as contributing to the health of body, mind and spirit. In āyurveda, the role of food as a major influence on the system is emphasised (as we literally take food into the body and it becomes part of us), and Desikachar often equated *tapas* specifically with dietary discipline. Whatever supports we adopt in our *tapas*, we should remember that *tapas* is always focused on the removal of something that is unwanted, unhelpful and ultimately an obstacle to our clarity, whether that be excess weight, lethargy, agitation, or unhelpful patterns of thought or behaviour. Modern yoga often emphasises purification of the body for our wellbeing. Traditional yoga emphasises purification of the body *and* the mind, for our 'well seeing': the cultivation of clarity and understanding.

6. *Rāja yoga* is usually understood to be the yoga of Patañjali, with its focus on various states of *samādhi*.

Svādhyāya: Developing our connection to the source

YS 2.44 svādhyāyād iṣṭa-devatā-saṃprayogaḥ

Through self-reflection a link with the chosen form of the divine is achieved

Svādhyāya is often translated as 'self-reflection'. It might be more literally translated as 'to approach the Self'. But which 'self' (*sva*) are we approaching and listening to? The relative one, with all its habits, prejudices, opinions and fickleness; or a deeper, still, quiet Self? Here we have linked the concept of *svādhyāya* to listening. In fact, one meaning of the word is 'the practice of chanting' – and this requires listening. Listening is also the most subtle and meditative of the five senses of knowing (*jñāna-indriya*). To really listen requires us to quieten down. In the context of *kriyā yoga*, we can think of *svādhyāya* as a gentle practice of quietening, listening, making space to hear ourselves. So, in contrast to the 'external support' we take with *tapas, svādhyāya* is about 'taking internal support seriously'. And as with *tapas*, this support is always there. Can we be still enough to listen to our deepest wisdom, and then committed enough to take support on it?

In the modern context, any activity that develops our self-awareness could be considered as *svādhyāya*. This could be our yoga practice, but it might also include counselling, other self-development activities, and the personal study of yoga and other subjects. The study of yoga philosophy can easily be seen as a peripheral activity in relation to the practice, but it is actually a very important aspect of our overall *sādhana* as it gives inspiration, helps to address areas of misunderstanding and, most importantly, provides food for reflection. Study for its own sake, as an intellectual exercise, is not *svādhyāya*. Study as a springboard for personal reflection and growth: this is a precious thing.

Embedded in the term *svādhyāya* is the verb meaning 'to go',[7] suggesting that self-enquiry is less a destination than a journey, directed towards the Self, *puruṣa*. In a traditional context, *svādhyāya* was connected with study of the sacred texts and chanting, as these dealt with the highest truths, i.e. the nature of the Self. Chanting was the means to both learn these texts and to make a heartfelt connection with their content. It was also associated with meditation and in particular the practice of *japa,* the recitation of a *mantra*, as this was also seen as a powerful means to approach the divine within us.

In the context of *kriyā yoga*, we can understand *svādhyāya* as arising from *tapas*. The effort required to observe our *tapas* and the responses it generates in us are an important source of personal reflection and learning. When everything is going well in our lives and there is no struggle, it is easy to become complacent, whereas it is often through personal challenges that we learn the most. While travelling in India, an ayurvedic doctor once told Dave that struggle was his friend and constant companion. This was said with true relish and enthusiasm, not as source of despair, and he is sure that this was the sense in which he meant it. He made a lasting impression and we remember his words often.

In a similar way, we can see *svādhyāya* as providing the raw material for *īśvara praṇidhāna*. Through self-reflection, we see more clearly the limits of our control. We might reflect upon our place within the larger scheme of things and better appreciate the scope of our lives within the sweep of history and human endeavour. *Īśvara praṇidhāna*, a surrender to the process of life and forces greater than ourselves, is fuelled by the reflections of *svādhyāya* if we can relate to our life's joys, challenges and limitations with acceptance and trust.

Svādhyāya and *niyama*

Svādhyāya is to *saṃtoṣa* as *tapas* is to *śauca*: it is the means to deepen *saṃtoṣa*. We have seen how *saṃtoṣa* arises from our

7. From the root *i*, to go.

inner connection, and *svādhyāya* is the practice to travel this inward path.

The fruit of *svādhyāya* given in the second chapter of the Yoga Sūtra can seem, at first, a little cryptic: "Through self-reflection a link with the chosen form of the divine (*iṣṭa devatā*) is achieved". *Iṣṭa devatā* is an important concept here: it represents the form through which one might relate to and approach the divine. This may be different for different people, hence the multitude of deities in the Indian tradition. It is accepted that to reach realisation of the highest principles, beyond conventional conceptual understanding, is difficult, and that deities with form and qualities are easier to relate to. Hence the traditional association with *japa*, the recitation of a mantra, which represents a connection to a particular form of the divine. Mantra are commonly associated with a particular deity, such as Śiva or Sarasvati. The repetition of mantra, practised as meditation with focus on the deity's qualities, and often accompanied with appropriate visualisation, is seen as the means to approach and make contact with that form of divine energy. Perhaps what is important to appreciate here is the metaphor of 'approaching and making contact with', reflected in the meaning of *svādhyāya* as 'moving towards' the Self. *Japa* and meditation on the form of a deity that has significant personal meaning, is seen as a powerful means to make this journey.

It is not essential to use a mantra associated with an Indian deity to embrace *svādhyāya*: any valid means to develop our self-awareness could be included. But it is important to understand some of the principles suggested if we want to go deeper. *Svādhyāya* represents a journey inwards, taken in the spirit of commitment and trust that something may be approached as a profound support, and which is beyond the limitations and frailties of our normal self (hence it is *devatā* – divine). *Svādhyāya* is an active process, something that we must engage in, but in contrast to *tapas* which concerns itself with the material, *svādhyāya* takes us inwards towards our inner experience of the sacred and ultimately the divine within us all.

We have suggested that *svādhyāya* is the means to cultivate *saṃtoṣa*. As our relationship to what carries us from inside deepens, we can develop a profound contentment from that. Such a contentment is not dependent on external circumstances: in fact, it allows us to be increasingly present with what is in our world with equanimity and openness, regardless of the form our lives take.

Sādhana: Vedic chanting as *kriyā yoga*

Vedic chanting emphasises the faithful and accurate reproduction of a text by a student exactly as taught by the teacher. The Vedic texts have been faithfully passed down and preserved by a long lineage of teachers and are precisely annotated to indicate their tonal structure. It obeys six distinct rules: the exact pronunciation of the Sanskrit sounds, the relative length of different syllables, the force of the pronunciation, the rhythm, melody (based on three notes), and continuity of the chant. Traditionally, there is no room for individual interpretation or improvisation and Krishnamacharya believed that through the disciplined and regular practice of Vedic chanting all the benefits of *kriyā yoga* can be achieved.

As we have already observed, chanting sacred texts is described by Vyāsa as an important form of *svādhyāya*. If we consider the components of *kriyā yoga* as categories which we can use to classify different practices, then clearly Vedic chanting is *svādhyāya*. However, we can also consider how the practice might embody aspects of all three limbs.

Chanting for twenty minutes or more in a very disciplined fashion can be intense. Taking a one-to-one chanting lesson for an hour can require a level of concentration that is often exhausting. In such a class, there is a constant requirement to really listen to the teacher and then attempt to reproduce what has been heard precisely. Additionally, the texts are in Sanskrit, which for many is unfamiliar, and many of the words and phrases can be long and complex. Traditionally Vedic chanting would be practised without a written text; this requires the student to pay even more attention to the recitation, and eventually to memorise it.

Chanting with such precision and within such strict rules sets boundaries that challenge us, making the practice a strong mental *tapas*. It can be both difficult and frustrating, but staying with it adds to the *tapas*. Chanting demands that we both use our breath in a controlled way and give the recitation some energy. This stimulates *agni*, the digestive fire. It is no wonder that it is common to feel ravenously hungry after intense Vedic chanting! We also feel different in some way, as if there has been a distinct energetic shift: the *tapas* of the practice transforms us on an energetic and psychological level.

The practice is a mirror, showing us how we respond to challenges, successes and frustrations. We begin to notice our patterns. This is one aspect of *svādhyāya* as self-reflection. To notice how we change and our minds fluctuate we need something stable: the rigour and structure of Vedic chanting provides such a stable support.

In a traditional sense also, the chanting of the sacred texts, which speak of the highest truths and the nature of the Self, leads us on a journey quite literally back to ourselves. In the Vedic tradition, the first point of learning was correct pronunciation, and there are many stories where the incorrect pronunciation of mantra or sacred passages leads to unwanted or adverse consequences.

As we begin to grapple with more complex passages and words (and in Sanskrit there can be some very long words and mind-bogglingly long lines), we begin to realise that the biggest obstacle is our own minds. Our anticipation of a difficulty and the tension that arises around it are often the limiting factors. Our hopes and fears, the desire to get it right and our feelings of self-worth all become mixed up. It can be a very emotive and deeply personal process. This is all part of the *svādhyāya*, but then the question arises: what can be done?

There comes a point in all such disciplines when we realise that there are limits to what we can achieve through determination and willpower alone. This is not to say that practice, *abhyāsa*, with all that implies, is not essential. But with *abhyāsa* there must be *vairāgya*. If *tapas* and *svādhyāya* are aspects of *abhyāsa*, *īśvara praṇidhāna* takes us towards *vairāgya*. Once we realise that the tightness and neurotic aspects of our own endeavour are limiting, maybe we can begin to let go, open up and trust in the process. This takes us into the realm of *īśvara praṇidhāna*.

The same journey can be explored with most of the practices of yoga. Although some fall more easily into a particular basket, most can be understood as embodying the three aspects of *kriyā yoga* if approached in the right way. Thus *kriyā yoga* not only becomes a template for the range of practices that we might engage in (to cover the three boxes), but also a template for our approach to each particular practice.

Chapter 14

स्वविषयासंप्रयोगे चित्तस्य स्वरूपानुकार
इवेन्द्रियाणां प्रत्याहारः ।

Guarding the Senses

YS 2.54 sva-viṣaya-asaṃprayoge cittasya sva-rūpānukara iva indriyāṇāṃ pratyāhāraḥ

'Withdrawing the senses' requires that we disengage them from their objects, so that they may follow the form of the mind's true nature instead

Pratyāhāra is the fifth of the eight limbs of yoga; it follows prāṇāyāma, and is the last topic in Chapter 2 of the Yoga Sūtra. It precedes the discussion of the 'inner limbs' (*dhāraṇā, dhyāna* and *samādhi*) that deal with the stages of meditation and which open Chapter 3. *Pratyāhāra* is a state of withdrawing the senses so that we are no longer distracted by external perceptions inconsistent with our direction of focus. When the focus is deeply inwards it may become temporarily unaware of external sensory events. The senses are described 'as if following the form of the mind,' which, in the highest state of *nirodha*, is very clear and still.

In his commentary, Vyāsa uses a beautiful image to describe the senses in *pratyāhāra*: they are like bees who follow, and rest with, the queen bee. The mind is the queen bee and the senses are her faithful servants who become still when their mistress is still. When the senses are at the service of the mind, we are able to choose where to 'place' them, rather than being controlled by them.

The state of the senses is an enduring topic of discussion throughout the Indian spiritual tradition. When uncontrolled they are like unruly horses that tug us this way and that, dragging the mind along with them. They therefore have to be restrained and taught who is boss. In Sanskrit the senses are called *indriya*, which indicates that they are (ideally) at the service of Indra, the Lord of the Gods. In this context, our 'Indra' is *puruṣa*, the transcendental Self. Our senses and mind[1] are thus in the service of *puruṣa*; the senses present us with experiences and the mind digests them.

According to the Yoga Sūtra, *pratyāhāra* is not a practice, but rather a state arising from our meditative focus. Prāṇāyāma is the primary means to cultivate this interiorised state. Investigating the nature of the senses, paying them conscious attention and using techniques that actively engage the senses are important means to engaging the mind, but are not technically *pratyāhāra*. However, they are very useful and are certainly part of the rich tapestry of yoga practice.

1. *Manas*, the part of the mind closest to the senses, is also referred to as one of the *indriya*.

The senses can lead us astray

The power of the senses has been acknowledged throughout the history of yoga. They are our interface to the world, the very means by which we experience reality. No wonder the senses and objects of sensual experience have such power over us.

Anything that can be experienced through the senses is termed *viṣaya*. This word is used for any object of the senses and often refers to an area of focus in meditation. The word *viṣaya* may be derived from the root *si*, meaning 'to bind', and thus a *viṣaya* is any object that in some sense binds us through the senses. In meditation, where we deliberately use a chosen direction of focus, this property can be useful. However, in daily life this 'binding' action of sensory objects can be unconscious and often unhelpful. A single chocolate can turn into half a dozen before you know it!

We have already met the *kleśa* – and *rāga* (desire) and *dveṣa* (aversion) in particular. Although desire and aversion are impulses in the mind, they relate to sensory experiences of the past. It is through our senses that our desires and fears are founded, and through them also that they can be subsequently fulfilled or thwarted. Although *duḥkha* (suffering) is a psychological phenomenon, the senses are almost always implicated, like accessories in a crime.

So, what is wrong with sensual experience? It is, after all, an important part of being human. The answer from this perspective is that nothing is wrong: it is the very thing that allows us to enjoy the richness of life. However, it is problematic when the senses lead us towards behaviours that have negative consequences, cause us suffering (even if not immediately) and distract us from, or undermine, what we are seeking to achieve. In Chapter 6 we met the *antarāya* of *avirati*, an overindulgence of the senses which is either an over-reliance on sensory stimulation or a situation where sensual experience pulls us away from our focus.

The role of the senses is to serve, not to lead

In the Upaniṣads there are a number of passages where the senses and vital energies of the body are described as *deva*, deities. In the Vedic tradition, the lord of the various deities is Indra, so the *indriya* (senses) are the powers (*deva*) that are at the service of Indra. In yoga there are ten, or sometimes eleven, *indriya*. The first five, the *jñāna indriya* (the senses of knowing – *jñāna*), are the five senses with which we are all familiar (hearing, touching, seeing, tasting and smelling). We could think of these as our 'inputs', the ways that we receive the world. The second five are our 'outputs', the way we act on the world and are known as *karma indriya* (the senses of action – *karma*). They are the 'organs' of speech, grasping, movement, procreation and excretion. Although these are also commonly translated as 'senses', it is better to think of the *karma indriya* as the 'instruments of action' – the instruments by which we have an impact on the world around us. We project speech, we hold and manipulate things, we move about, we create children and we excrete, leaving various deposits! Sometimes the mind, or at least the aspect of the mind which coordinates and reasons (*manas*), is included as an eleventh instrument.

We are left with the question of who, or what, is the Indra which the *indriya* should serve. Who is the lord of our domain? The conventional answer is the mind, as it is the mind that decides where we will focus when we consciously direct the senses. However, in the philosophy of yoga, it is *puruṣa* that is the ultimate source of consciousness and thus we should consider Indra here to refer to *puruṣa*. The *indriya* (and the mind) are ultimately at the service of the Self (*puruṣa*), to present experience for a journey of awakening. From a practical point of view, however, we can say that the senses should be at the service of the mind, and the mind is then in the service of the Self. We must be masters of our senses rather than their slaves.

In the *Kaṭha Upaniṣad* we find a very famous metaphor of the chariot driven by the charioteer and carrying a warrior into battle. The horses are the senses (*indriya*), the reins are the mind (*manas*), the charioteer is the discerning faculty of the mind (*buddhi*), and the warrior is the Self (*puruṣa*). If uncontrolled, the horses pull against each other and take the chariot along a random path, dragging the reins with them. But if the charioteer is strong and accomplished, he uses the reins to control the horses so that they pull together and take the chariot in the desired direction. The warrior ultimately directs the charioteer to steer their course. In a similar way, the Self can be taken on a wild uncontrolled ride through life, or, if everything is at its service, the journey of life can be directed where it needs to go.

Becoming aware of the senses

Yoga teaches the cultivation of awareness of all aspects of our lives. This requires us to become increasingly conscious of how we function, and this naturally includes the senses. We spend much of our lives on autopilot, often preoccupied with thoughts of one thing, while doing another. Although our senses are functioning at some level all the time, we are unaware of much of what is being presented to us and indeed, the effect it has upon us. We are masters of filtering out unwanted familiar sensory input. City dwellers sleep soundly next to busy roads. Ironically when visiting the quiet of the country, they may be disturbed by the early morning cockerel that their country hosts no longer even 'hear'. This automatic pilot and filtering function allows us to focus on what is essential, but it comes at a price: it can deaden us to the richness that our sensory life has to offer.

There is a well-known mindfulness exercise in which participants are invited to eat a raisin.[2] They pretend to have arrived from another planet where there are no raisins, and encounter it for the first time. They take time to examine and feel the raisin's shape and texture, and then eat it as

2. From Jon Kabat-Zinn MBSR course.

consciously as possible, giving time to feel it in their mouths and allowing its flavour to unfold and fully develop. Taking time to really notice what our senses come into contact with can open up a whole new panorama of sensual experience that we normally miss. This is a simple way to bring more colour and joy into many aspects of our lives, while also creating conditions where we are focused and fully present.

Engaging the senses

When we focus on our sensory experiences they can have a magnetic effect on our minds. Unexpected stimuli, such as a sudden noise, can pull us sharply away from our point of focus, and easily create distraction and disturbance. However, we can also use the pull of the senses consciously in our practice to help us engage. In fact, using the senses on all levels has been a strong feature of many Indian rituals and meditative practices: chanting, bells and drums feed the ears, incense feeds the sense of smell, elaborate forms and symbols (whether real or visualised) feed our eyes, and ritual gestures feed our sense of touch.

In our regular āsana practice, the more we cultivate our felt sense, as we move into, hold or move out of postures, the more deeply engaged we become. The use of *bhāvana* (specific feelings or ideas to cultivate, imagine and feel), employs this very process where we combine something imagined with something real that can be 'felt'. We deliberately cultivate a two-way interaction between the mind and the senses in order to deepen and refresh our experiences.

In this particular tradition, we often use sound as a means to enhance the power of an āsana. Simple sounds are often best, such as a sustained *ā* sound in, for example, a standing forward bend. The sound directly engages the senses of hearing and feeling (we feel the vibration as well as hear it), and we cannot help but be drawn into the whole experience. It also requires us to commit something of ourselves in a way that doing the posture silently may not require, and it touches us emotionally in a manner that can be quite unexpected. After all, on the surface, bending forwards making the sound *ā*, is nothing profound. But in reality, directly engaging the senses through both making and receiving sound can touch us deeply. It can act as a shortcut to the very core of our being.

Bringing the senses under control

We have seen how the senses can lead us astray. We have also seen how investigating the senses and using them to support our engagement in practice can be a very beneficial journey. However, as our practice becomes more inwards in focus there is more of a need to temper the senses because they can easily pull us outwards once again. The *Bhagavad Gītā* famously advises the *yogin* to withdraw the senses as a tortoise withdraws its limbs.[3]

Generally, unless we are consciously using the senses as a support (e.g. sound in āsana), we seek to minimise the distractions that the senses might cause. Ideally, the space where we practise should be clear, uncluttered and relatively quiet. On a very practical level, we advise that the eyes are kept closed except when sight is useful for maintaining balance. Similarly, we advise new group-class students to try to avoid looking around the room and becoming distracted by their fellow students, to avoid talking and to remain as self-contained as possible, even if there are outside distractions. Once students know basically what they are doing, we tend to instruct with minimal demonstration. We want them to inhabit their own practice with as little outside sensory input as possible.

Pratyāhāra as the fifth of the eight limbs

Patañjali lists *pratyāhāra*, the withdrawal of the senses, as the fifth of the eight limbs of yoga. It is the last of the 'outer' limbs, and prior to the three 'inner' limbs which

3. *Bhagavad Gītā* 2.58.

deal with the process of meditation and the mind itself. If we consider the eight limbs as ordered from outer to inner, *pratyāhāra* marks the interface between the external world of relationships, body and breath, to the inner world of the mind. Whereas the activity of the senses usually takes our attention outwards, through *pratyāhāra,* our attention is contained within, opening the door to inner experience.

The word *pratyāhāra* derives from the root *hṛ* meaning 'to withdraw' or 'lead away', with the prefixes *prati* and *ā* indicating the opposite to their usual direction of travel (so inwards, rather than outwards). Alternatively, the word may be seen as comprising *prati* + *āhāra*, where *āhāra* is food, and therefore *pratyāhāra* is where the senses are led away from their usual 'food' – the world and its objects that can be 'eaten' by the senses.

Pratyāhāra is not a state that is required or even recommended during daily life. It is desirable only during the meditative journey where we are seeking to direct the mind inwards and we wish to prevent the mind's usual tendency to follow the senses and their outward connections. This is important to appreciate, lest we consider the senses as enemies to be permanently overcome. They have an essential role in allowing us to navigate, experience and act in the world.

Pratyāhāra is sometimes described as the forgotten practice in yoga and students ask if there are specific practices for *pratyāhāra*. It is misleading to say that there are *pratyāhāra* practices as such. The key to *pratyāhāra* is to understand that in a state when the mind is directed inwards (or is very still), the senses follow the mind, and so *pratyāhāra* is a *consequence* of the state of the mind. As we have seen, Vyāsa reinforces this with the image of the bees (the senses) following their queen (the mind) so that when the queen rests, they rest also and thus disengage from their usual objects. When the mind withdraws from its normal activity, the senses follow and 'other means for mastery of the senses are unnecessary'.[4] As Desikachar puts

4. Vyāsa in his commentary to YS 2.55.

it, "it is very difficult to find a technique for the practice of *pratyāhāra* itself, because the more we use the senses the more they focus on their objects. All we can do is create a condition in which the senses lose their habitual significance and only help the mind in the state of *dhyāna*."[5]

This situation would apparently put *pratyāhāra* as a consequence of the limbs that follow it (*dhāraṇā*, *dhyāna* and *samādhi*). This is true in some sense, and is why we must be careful not to see the eight limbs as simply a linear order of practices. However, as we have stated, the tradition maintains that the practice that really cultivates the inner focus encouraging the state of *pratyāhāra* is, in fact, its preceding limb, prāṇāyāma. Prāṇāyāma has a special role in pacifying the habitually turbulent nature of the mind, and thereby stabilises the senses.

The final sūtra of the second chapter describes the fruit of *pratyāhāra*: the highest state of *pratyāhāra,* which gives complete control of the senses. Vyāsa reaffirms that through one-pointedness of mind, the senses naturally disconnect from their objects and this indeed is *pratyāhāra*. It is interesting that Vyāsa also lists a series of other understandings of *pratyāhāra* that he emphatically refutes, in the context of the *aṣṭāṅga* yoga system at least. These alternative views define *pratyāhāra* as follows:

- non-attachment to objects of the senses that lead one away from the path of yoga
- avoiding sensual indulgence prohibited by the sacred texts
- consciously choosing to engage the senses rather than being a slave to them
- absence of attachment or aversion to sensual experiences which might lead to distress

All of these seem sensible to varying degrees, but what is important to appreciate here is the specific technical meaning given to *pratyāhāra* in the Yoga Sūtra: where the mind is stable and internally focused, resulting in the

5. *Religiousness in Yoga* p. 183.

withdrawal of the senses from external stimuli. As Vyāsa also states, in such a situation no other means for guarding the senses are necessary, as the senses are following their true master. Rather than applying external constraints or disciplines, the activity of the senses has been temporarily suspended at source.

Sādhana: Minimising distractions, engaging the senses, resting the senses

Patañjali's definition of *pratyāhāra* as a state arising from a profound one-pointedness of mind makes it potentially difficult to achieve. In practice, we are often more concerned with the habitual functioning of the senses and their role in directing the mind. There are some simple practical things that we do to either minimise their distracting influences, or alternatively to engage the senses positively.

The simplest example of reducing sensory distraction is to close the eyes during the practice when it is appropriate. This acknowledges the strong pull of visual stimuli that draw us out into the world and away from ourselves. In āsana we use a simple rule of thumb: *eyes open for standing, and closed for everything else*. In standing postures the eyes are useful for maintaining balance, but even in standing, for the simplest of movements where balance is not important, closing the eyes can be beneficial. This can transform the practice for new students: as soon as the eyes are closed for a couple of postures, a new inner focus and calm arises.

In teaching group classes, the most dramatic example of the difference between eyes open and closed is often in a seated twist (fig 14.1) where the spine is rotated and the head turned as if looking over one shoulder.

Because of the turning of the head, new students commonly keep their eyes open and gaze over their shoulder to the edges of the room. The posture remains a very outer

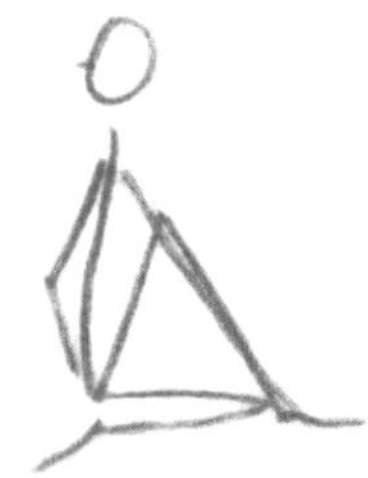

fig 14.1

experience and this is often marked by distraction and fidgeting when the posture is completed. The seated twist is essentially an inner, meditative posture where the attention is held within, in the central axis between the head and sacrum. If the posture is initiated, maintained and completed with eyes closed, this inner focus is supported and the effect on the student is noticeably different. This is just one example, but the principle holds in many postures particularly where they lend themselves to less movement and longer periods of stay.

In some traditions, by contrast, the visual sense is actively engaged during āsana (and sometimes prāṇāyāma) through deliberate 'gazing' at key points in the body. By binding the visual sense to a single point, the focus of the mind is supported. In this approach, although we don't tend to use gazing so frequently, we often use sound as a deliberate means to engage the senses. As we have already discussed, bending forwards while making a simple sound for the duration of the movement can be very useful on many levels. It is an obvious means to encourage a long and full exhale (you have to exhale to make the sound), but it is also a very sensual experience that engages the voice, hearing and feeling as we experience the vibrations in our body. It also requires a level of engagement and commitment in a way that is quite different from breathing alone. We can be both engaged strongly through the senses and touched deeply, and using sound can be an emotional experience for many students.

Finally, there are some techniques that directly attempt to reduce the external sensory inputs and encourage us to reorientate internally. An example of this would be *śaṇmukhī mudrā* where the 'gateways' into the head are symbolically closed:

- the middle and forefinger of each hand cover the eyes
- ring fingers symbolically block the nasal passages (although placed alongside the nostrils, the fingers do not interfere with the breathing)
- little fingers touch the sides of the closed mouth
- thumbs literally close the ears.

The elbows are held at shoulder height and the posture is maintained for a minute or so. This can lead to tension in the shoulders and neck, and so we need to slowly develop our capacity for comfortably staying in the posture over a period of time. The experience is interesting in that it is very interiorising, leaving the practitioner feeling somehow more centred and sensually rested. It also brings a freshness to the senses, and particularly to the sense of hearing. Krishnamacharya felt that this was a very useful practice.[6]

For most of us, the vastly dominant sense is that of sight, since the majority of our understanding of the world comes from what we can see. A modified version of *śaṇmukhī mudrā* which addresses only the eyes, is the technique of palming. Here, the heel of the hand rests lightly at the base of the eye socket, and the fingers are up over the hairline. The eyes themselves are closed and rest in the middle of the palm. This can be done very effectively in both seated and lying positions and has the added benefit that it does not build up tension in the neck and shoulders in the same way. It is also easy to practise dynamically, or even asymmetrically where we cover first one eye, and then the other.

6. Krishnamacharya recommended the practice for five minutes, which is actually quite a long time to keep the arms raised. In practice, we often do a round of about one minute, followed by simple sitting for 30 seconds to a minute, repeated two or three times.

Chapter 15

त्रयमेकत्र संयमः।

Exploring the Potential of the Mind

YS 3.4 trayam ekatra saṃyamaḥ

When the three stages of meditation are practised together as a single process, this is saṃyama

The process of meditation is described by the three inner limbs, *dhāraṇā*, *dhyāna* and *samādhi*. These three steps describe a process and should be considered as a continuum rather than as discrete or separate practices. When they come together as one, this process of meditative absorption is known as *saṃyama*, literally 'complete restraint' of the mind. This is consistent with the understanding of *nirodha* as 'directing the mind in a chosen direction and restraining (*nirodha*) all activities of the mind (*citta vṛtti*) that are contrary to that direction.' Although this may appear to be a very rigid controlled process, it is actually a delicate play between *abhyāsa* and *vairāgya*, requiring a high level of *vairāgya*.

Dhāraṇā is the first step in the process and is defined in YS 3.1 as 'binding the mind to a single place (*deśa*)'. The essential quality of *dhāraṇā* is the intention to link the mind to a chosen object or a field of enquiry. In *dhāraṇā* the link with the *deśa* is stable, and the attention is focused.

The second of the inner limbs, *dhyāna*, is characterised by a deepening connection to the field of enquiry so that we start to gain new insight. In *dhyāna* our perceptions and mental responses link up with a new level of coherence and freshness. *Dhyāna* is characterised both by the *citta vṛtti* flowing towards the *deśa* (indicating the stability of the link), and also by their return to the mind (facilitating new insight or perception).

The pinnacle of the meditative process, and the last of the eight limbs, is *samādhi* (literally 'putting together completely'). There are two basic levels of 'yogic' *samādhi* and it is the first, *sabīja samādhi,* that is being referred to here (the other is *nirbīja samādhi*). *Sabīja samādhi* is directed meditation (i.e. a meditation in which there is an object or field of enquiry), while *nirbīja samādhi* does not require an object.[1]

Patañjali defines *sabīja samādhi* as having two key characteristics. The first is that the essential nature of the object of meditation shines forth, implying that this is an extraordinary level of perception and that the object fills the mind. The second follows from this: that for the duration of the *samādhi,* it is as if any sense of separation between meditator and object of meditation disappears, and there is a feeling of 'oneness'. The sūtra emphasises that this is an 'as if' experience, so it only lasts for the duration of the *samādhi*.

Saṃyama is when *dhāraṇā, dhyāna* and *samādhi* become one deep, seamless process. The traditional commentators explain that *saṃyama* is the process of meditation practised with the same object in mind for a long period of time. This creates a habitual pattern for the mind (*saṃskāra*) that allows the meditator to achieve an extraordinary level of insight with respect to the object of enquiry. This is said to be the realm of true wisdom (YS 3.5). It is from such a deep level of meditative enquiry that the 'special powers' (*siddhi*) arise. These powers form a large part of Chapter 3 of the Yoga Sūtra, and are the most extensive topic within the text.[2]

1. *Sabīja samādhi* is synonymous with *ekāgra*, and *nirbīja samadhi* is synonymous with *niruddha* as discussed in Chapter 2.

2. Amounting to 40 sūtras within a total of 55 in Chapter 3 alone, and 195 across the whole of the Yoga Sūtra.

Yoga is meditation and meditation is the key to developing wisdom

Yoga is *samādhi*, according to Vyāsa is his commentary to the very first sūtra (YS 1.1). In YS 3.4 we are introduced to a new term, *saṃyama* – the culmination of the meditative process described by the three final limbs of the eight limbs of yoga: *dhāraṇā*, *dhyāna* and *samādhi*. Breaking this down into three separate terms is for the convenience of explanation only: in truth, the meditative process is continuous and may not even involve all three 'limbs' – indeed *samādhi* may be something that we never or rarely experience. But Patañjali defines *saṃyama* as the process of meditation where all the three steps are present together 'as one'. He presents this as the route to gaining insight and wisdom, and thereby gaining certain mastery or control. The yoga tradition is full of stories of yogis who have extraordinary powers (*siddhi*), such as the ability to become invisible, to float in the air or travel great distances almost instantly.

Whether or not we believe such claims, meditation is clearly seen as the route to developing insight into the nature of things, and ultimately, into the nature of ourselves. When the mind is honed to focus with total clarity and lack of projection, our potential for insight is extraordinary. This is something we can all readily experience: in quiet moments when the mind is uncluttered and clear, new and profound insights arise.

A typical yoga class consists largely of āsana, perhaps with ten minutes of prāṇāyāma, and little, if any, seated meditation. And yet, according to Vyāsa, yoga *is* meditation and Patañjali himself defines yoga as '*citta vṛtti nirodha*' in YS 1.2. If we are serious about pursuing yoga in the spirit of the Yoga Sūtra, we should therefore consider the significance of seated meditation practice.

Our training in this tradition has undoubtedly focused on the practice of āsana and prāṇāyāma, with much less emphasis on seated meditation. But does the meditative process apply only to formal seated meditation, or can it apply to the other practices such as āsana and prāṇāyāma as well? In both āsana and prāṇāyāma the principle intention is to engage the mind and our approach has been to make the meditative engagement of the mind the most important aspect. We are not suggesting that āsana and prāṇāyāma replace seated meditation practices, but that they can *also* be meditative practices in which the basic principles, and those of the 'inner limbs', can apply.

Saṃyama is explained by Vyāsa as the process of deep meditation (*dhāraṇā*, *dhyāna* and *samādhi*) towards the same object of enquiry over a long period – weeks, months or even years. The *siddhi* imply complete knowledge of something which leads to its mastery. This requires that

'In both āsana and prāṇāyāma, the principle intention is to engage the mind.'

it is explored fully 'from all sides'.[3] Time and repeated practice are necessary. The Yoga Sūtra states that the mind works through habitual patterns (*saṃskāra*), well-worn grooves that we can slot into with ease. Many of these are unconscious and indeed unhelpful in our lives. But *saṃskāra* can also be helpful. Krishnamacharya stated that yoga practice itself is a *saṃskāra*. We should understand that meditation is also a *saṃskāra*; in short, it gets easier with practice.

We can apply the principles of *saṃyama* to many areas of life. Observation in teaching yoga can have something of the spirit of *saṃyama*. A teacher who brings this meditative quality to the observation of their students can achieve extraordinary levels of perception – as we have experienced ourselves with our teachers. A highly skilled and experienced surgeon could also be an example of someone who has a *siddhi* resulting from dedicated *saṃyama,* focused practice and study in a specific area over a long period of time resulting in extraordinary knowledge and mastery.

3. Reflecting the idea of *paridṛṣṭa* discussed in Chapter 10 with respect to prāṇāyāma.

In Chapter 3 of the Yoga Sūtra, Patañjali lists many possibilities for *saṃyama* and its fruits. Although this part of the Yoga Sūtra can seem somewhat opaque, even bizarre, and the list of different *saṃyama* and their fruits rather random, there is an internal logic. The list mirrors the evolutionary structure of the world as proposed by the Sāṃkhya system.[4] Sāṃkhya, as we discussed in Chapter 7, is the sister philosophy to yoga and provides a foundation for understanding the world.[5] Sāṃkhya proposes a system that classifies the world into twenty-five essential principles (*tattva*) and many of the *siddhi* can be understood as the result of mastering these principles.

Dhāraṇā: Stabilising the link

YS 3.1 deśa bandhaḥ cittasya dhāraṇā

Dhāraṇā involves binding the mind to a place or location

In *dhāraṇā*, we focus the mind on a chosen object or field of enquiry (*deśa*) and maintain that link for some time. This requires intention and effort. The word *dhāraṇā* comes from the Sanskrit root *dhṛ* meaning 'to hold' or 'support'; the very word itself implies an intention to hold the object of focus. It is often translated as 'concentration', although this carries with it unhelpful associations of hard work and a furrowed brow. For *dhāraṇā* to evolve to the next level, *dhyāna*, such tightness is counterproductive and actually blocks the process it is trying to facilitate.

Dhāraṇā: *Vṛtti* are focused and the mind is stable

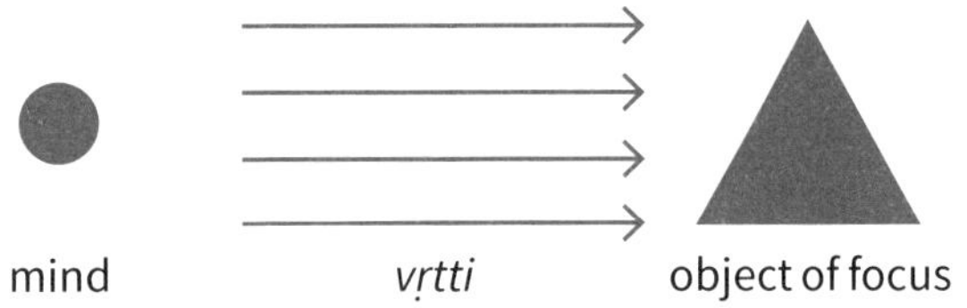

Many people are put off meditation because they feel that they cannot do it and fail when they try. They cannot

4. A discussion of *Sāṃkhya* and the evolution of the *tattva* is beyond the scope of this book but we would encourage the interested reader to explore this further. For a simple overview, see *The Funky Guru: Sāṃkhyārtha Saṃgraha: Essential Samkhya for Yoga Students* (Sadhana Mala publications).

5. The Yoga Sūtra assumes knowledge of the Sāṃkhya worldview.

maintain focus for any length of time, let alone 'empty' their minds (perhaps one of the least helpful instructions for anyone trying to meditate). Meditation involves *vinyāsa krama*: it is a gradual process. We should approach it with compassion towards ourselves and our unsteady minds, accepting that movement in the mind is natural and not something intrinsically bad. Training the mind is a little like training a puppy: it requires great patience and a firm, kind guiding hand. Repetition is key, coming back to the practice without anger and frustration, but with an even-handed persistence.

In most classes and workshops, insufficient attention is given to seriously maintaining focus. Although students know that it is part of the practice, it easily becomes secondary to the physicality and feel-good factor that the practice can bring. But *dhāraṇā* requires diligence and persistence, and is applicable to all aspects of the practice, not just formal meditation. *Dhāraṇā* requires us to switch on, not switch off, and this is an active process necessitating intention, effort and vigilance towards all the subtle attitudes and judgements that we bring to the process. It is almost inevitable that at some point our attitude will become too tight: it is a fine line between too much effort and too little.

It is easy to feel frustrated when we find it difficult to stop the mind from flitting from here to there. But it's worth remembering that because the mind is nothing but *guṇa,* and their nature is dynamic: it is only natural for the mind to move. In YS 3.9, Patañjali states that the mind has two possibilities: that of 'emergence' (*vyutthāna*) and that of 'stillness' (*nirodha*). Emergence is defined as any state of mind in which there are *vṛtti* (ideas, thoughts, feelings and memories) that rise up and become visible. What is less obvious, however, is that even in a state of *nirodha* there is actually movement, albeit more subtle and therefore less perceptible. The mind *appears* static in *nirodha* because there is the appearance of only one *vṛtti* (or image) but in fact, it is a continuous repetition of a single image – like a number of still frames of the same shot in a film. Both of these states, *vyutthāna* and *nirodha,* are largely habitual (they are *saṃskāra*), and so the more we practise, the more easily we can train our minds to focus peacefully – and thereby move from *vyutthāna* to *nirodha*. It is a matter of gradual and gentle training.

Although *dhāraṇā* requires us to have an intention to 'bind' or 'hold' the mind and to keep our attention stable, this is only the starting point. *Dharma* (which comes from same root *dhṛ* as *dhāraṇā*) is a complex word simply summed up as 'our purpose and responsibilities in life'. In the *Bhagavad Gītā,* following and fulfilling our *dharma* is considered a route to the highest yoga. There is a reciprocal relationship between a person and their *dharma*: if someone can 'hold' their *dharma* – follow their path diligently and fulfil their obligations – then their *dharma* will 'hold' them. Initially we actively carry our *dharma,* but then it begins to carry us: to take support on something, we must give support to it. This is a very helpful way to think about our relationship towards a *deśa*, which is effectively a support for our mind.

During *dhāraṇā* we begin by actively holding our attention towards the *deśa*, 'binding the mind'. But in order to allow the *deśa* to fully act as a support, we must relax and open our mind to become receptive. This takes us into the realm of *dhyāna*, but it comes from the attitude which we bring to *dhāraṇā*. The single direction arrows in the diagram, representing the stable focus of all mental activity towards the *deśa,* are really only the starting point for *dhāraṇā*. Peter Hersnack described how as the object of meditation deepens, the object can become 'guru'. Here the word has an interesting double meaning: both 'heavy' and also 'teacher'. On the one hand, the gravitational pull of the object increases (it becomes heavy) so that it both begins to hold us and increasingly fills our consciousness with its nature and qualities. But also, we learn something new and we are changed; the object functions like a teacher or *guru*.

The interplay between actively holding the mind's focus and allowing it to be receptive is like the *abhyāsa* and *vairāgya* of meditation. If we hold on to the object too tightly and intently, there is a danger that we simply project our existing associations and concepts onto it. There is no space for the reality of the object to touch us. However, if the link with the object is stable, and we allow ourselves to let go of expectations and preconceptions, the mind may open up to what is actually there.

Deśa is also a concept that requires some careful explanation. *Deśa* is literally 'a place' and in Vyāsa's commentary examples are given that are locations, in the body, such as the navel or the tip of the nose. The word is also used in the sūtra on prāṇāyāma (YS 2.50), and similarly refers to a physical location: the location where the breath is experienced in the body. However, the examples of *saṃyama* given in Chapter 3 of the Yoga Sūtra are much more diverse and not limited to physical locations. *Deśa* may be any focal point for the mind, including objects of meditation such as the breath itself, a mantra, a visualisation of the sun or even a deity, a question for contemplation, a physical or imagined symbol. There are endless possibilities.

The word is etymologically linked to the Sanskrit root *diś*, meaning 'to point'. From this perspective, *deśa* is that which points to something beyond itself, like a road sign to a nearby town. Many traditional objects of meditation, such as sacred symbols, mantra and even deity visualisations are *deśa* in this sense: they invite the meditator towards a reality or truth that is greater than the symbol itself.

Dhyāna: Deepening the link

YS 3.2 tatra pratyayaikatānatā dhyānam

From that (dhāraṇā), our perceptions become continuous and integrate: this is dhyāna

If we were to choose a single Sanskrit equivalent to the English word 'meditation' it would be *dhyāna*. *Dhyāna* comes from the Sanskrit root *dhyā*, meaning 'to think about' or 'contemplate'. In Sanskrit literature, *dhyāna* is used to refer to both meditation and also the culmination of the meditative process particularly in texts predating the Yoga Sūtra. *Samādhi* is a newer term used in the Yoga Sūtra, texts of a similar age, and subsequent texts.

In Patañjali's sequence of 'inner limbs', *dhyāna* refers to the deepening of the meditative process. It is a two-way process whereby the attention is maintained towards the object of meditation and something is received from it. In *dhyāna*, it is as if the object communicates something of itself to us and we begin to gain insight into its true nature.

Dhyāna: As involvement deepens, new insights arise

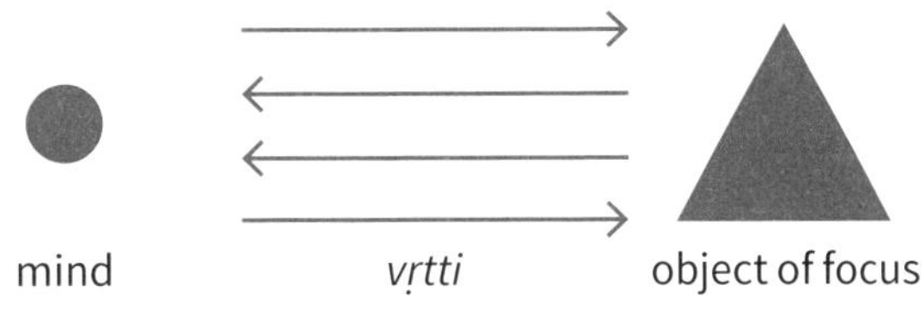

The word *tatra* in YS 3.2 means 'there', and it refers us back to the previous sūtra and the state of *dhāraṇā*. *Dhyāna* follows from the foundation of *dhāraṇā*. The defining feature of *dhyāna* is indicated by the phrase *pratyaya eka tānatā* which describes a particular state of the *pratyaya*, the ideas that arise in the mind in response to the meditation.

Pratyaya is a word that comes from the root *i* meaning 'to go', with a prefix *prati* that indicates a reversal or return. Thus, *pratyaya* are ideas that arise in the mind in response to 'a going and a coming back' (hence the arrows in both directions in our diagram). In the yogic view of perception there is a movement of *prāṇa* outwards towards an object of perception and a return movement of *prāṇa* carrying an impression or perception. In *dhyāna,* the *pratyaya* are said to be *eka tānatā*; they create a single continuity or interconnection.

Vyāsa understands the *eka tānatā* to be the continuity of the connection with the object. Whereas in *dhāraṇā* there is stability, but also the possibility of interruption, in *dhyāna* the link is continuous and not subject to distraction or interruption. *Dhāraṇā* is analogous to a stream of water droplets with small spaces between each droplet, whereas in *dhyāna* the flow of attention is continuous like pouring oil or honey.

There is another dimension to *eka tānatā* which is more related to the connection between the ideas that arise in the mind. Usually our perception of things is distorted and overlaid by assumptions, memories and expectations. Peter Hersnack referred to this as "the imperialism of meaning". Rather than impose our beliefs on the world – as an imperial or colonial power might – in *dhyāna,* our *pratyaya* begin to connect up in new ways that reflect the reality of what we are encountering. Our insights and perceptions become more consistent with the singular reality of the object in the here and now: *eka tānatā.*

The practice of meditation is not like travelling towards a destination through a tunnel. It evolves organically, with moments of focus, moments of receptivity, maybe something akin to a new insight and lots of drifting around with obscure peripheral thoughts. Lots of distraction, lots of reconnecting. Don't be concerned if you don't appear to be 'getting anywhere'. Even at this level, the concepts of *dhāraṇā* and *dhyāna* have a crucial role to play.

When meditating, Desikachar said he always made sure to have a pencil and notepad in his shirt pocket. As the mind settles, it is as if the threshold between conscious and unconscious thought becomes more permeable and all kinds of small insights, ideas or useful thoughts can arise. This peripheral bubbling of the mind can be both a distraction and a source of inspiration and insight, so we should acknowledge it as a common feature of the conversation that is *dhyāna*.

Samādhi: The connection becomes complete

YS 3.3 tadeva artha mātra nirbhāsam svarūpa śūnyamiva samādhiḥ

When the true nature of the object reveals itself,
and fills the mind as if we are no longer present,
that is samādhi

The culmination of the meditative process is called *samādhi*. The first word, *tadeva*, means 'there/that indeed' and links to the previous sūtra concerning *dhyāna*. *Samādhi* arises out of *dhyāna* and can be understood as a particular state of *dhyāna*, rather than something completely different. As we have said, prior to the Yoga Sūtra, the term *dhyāna* was used to describe the highest states of meditation and it is only after the Yoga Sūtra that the term *samādhi* became more widely used.

Samādhi: Total identification with object leads to complete understanding

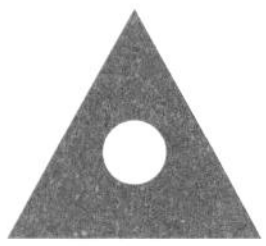

Samādhi means 'to go into', 'go together', 'put together' or be 'deeply rooted'. In *samādhi* we go into the object of meditation fully, become totally absorbed in it, and everything in our understanding and experience of the

object becomes complete. The mind is deeply rooted and stable. Patanjali defines *samādhi* more specifically in YS 3.3 by describing two fundamental conditions that apply.

The first concerns the phrase *artha mātra nirbhāsam*, 'the essential nature of the object alone shines forth'. In *samādhi* our comprehension and insight become complete and this illuminates the mind so that nothing else is present.

The second, *svarūpa śūnyam iva* means 'as if empty of our own form'. This follows as a consequence of the first and refers to the experience of losing our sense of separateness from the object of meditation. This state lasts only as long as *samādhi* – from a few fleeting moments to longer, sustained periods for more advanced yogis.

Keeping in mind these two conditions – deep absorption and the loss of any sense of separateness – is the key to understanding the meaning of *samādhi* in the Yoga Sūtra.

Two levels of *samādhi*

As we explored in Chapter 2, Vyāsa presents five states of mind. The first three are:

- obsessively active (*kṣipta*) – characterised by an excess of rajas
- dull and passive (*mūḍha*) – characterised by an excess of tamas
- clear but unstable (*vikṣipta*) – characterised by instability

These states all have the potential for a 'sort of' *samādhi* – that is, a type of absorption. We can be truly absorbed in our obsessive activity (excess *rajas*), or stuck in dullness (excess *tamas*). And we may have moments of insight (*sattva*) when we are in the third state (*vikṣipta*), but the state is fickle. Because *sattva* does not dominate, and there is no stability, none of these is a **yoga** *samādhi*; they are like false *samādhi*.

Vyāsa does go on to elaborate two further states, which *are* yoga *samādhi*: *ekāgra* and *niruddha*. In the first, we focus on an object of meditation; it is therefore *sabīja* ('with seed'). In the second, there is no external object of support and the state is thus called *nirbīja,* 'without seed'. In Chapter 1 of the Yoga Sūtra, Patañjali directly refers to these two levels, which he calls *saṃprajñāta* and *anya* ('the other one') respectively.

YS 1.17 vitarka vicāra ānanda asmitārūpa anugamāt saṃprajñātaḥ

Saṃprajñāta samādhi has four levels: discursive thought, subtle insight, bliss and identification

Saṃprajñāta, the first level of *samādhi,* is 'with seed' and even here there is a hierarchy – one state of *samādhi* evolves into the next (*anugamāt*). Its four levels, *vitarka, vicāra, ānanda* and *asmitārūpa* are complex technical terms in this context, but we can understand them in a simple way as each being a more subtle form of *samādhi* than its precursor. In *vitarka* there is a comprehension of the gross form of the object of contemplation and this is accompanied by some discursive thought. It is looking at the object from various angles. This evolves into *vicāra,* where we see something of the hidden depths of an object, aspects which are not apparent initially. *Vicāra* thus takes us to a deeper comprehension of an object. With this evolves a feeling of joy (*ānanda*); our minds are profoundly contented as they are focused, engaged and working at their optimal level. As a result of this process, our sense of self shifts away from our constructed self (*asmitā kleśa*) towards the simplicity and truth of the feeling of simply being alive and aware (*asmitā rūpa*). We could see this deepening of the process of *samādhi* as a sort of 'subtle form of *saṃyama*': just as *dhāraṇā* evolves into *dhyāna* and then *samādhi,* so *vitarka* evolves into *vicāra* and then to *ānanda* and finally *asmitā rūpa.*[6]

6. The various traditional commentators generally agree that the different levels of *saṃprajñāta* involve focusing on increasingly subtle levels of objects. However, for simplicity, we have presented this process as increasingly refined levels of *samādhi* arising from the same object.

YS 1.18 virāmapratyaya abhyāsapūrvaḥ saṃskāraśeṣaḥ anyaḥ

The other (level of samādhi), arising from the practice of the previous level, is a state in which only subtle psychological patterns remain: thoughts and ideas have temporarily ceased

Although Patañjali rather cryptically refers to the second level of yoga *samādhi* as *anya* (other), Vyāsa more explicitly calls it *asaṃprajñāta.* This state follows from the practice of the other (*abhyāsa-pūrvaḥ*) and is akin to the *nirbīja* state where there is no external object of contemplation. It is an extremely rarefied state; because there is no external object, the consciousness of *puruṣa* is only aware of itself. All other *vṛtti* or activities of the mind have ceased and the mind is like a flawless jewel. Vyāsa states that it arises from extensive practice of *saṃprajñāta samādhi* with increasingly subtle supports for our meditation (i.e. objects), accompanied by the highest levels of *vairāgya.*[7] It is a state of pure being and is considered the pinnacle of the Yogic path.

Although it is of little practical relevance for the majority of us struggling with our practice in everyday life, it is nevertheless essential to be aware of *asaṃprajñāta* (or *nirbīja*) *samādhi.* Without an appreciation of the two levels of *samādhi,* it is easy to become confused about the teachings of the Yoga Sūtra and its commentaries, which discuss both levels. *Nirbīja samādhi* is something that may arise through advanced practice, but cannot be practised in the ordinary sense of the word as it is not possible to simply 'stop the activity of the mind' by an act of will. It's worth re-emphasising – trying to 'stop the mind' in meditation is one of the most unhelpful instructions that anyone can give! Our *sādhana* should be to direct, rather than to stop, the mind.

7. Vyāsa emphasises the need for the highest form of *vairāgya* (as described in YS 1.16) as the most important factor for cultivating *asaṃprajñāta samādhi.* The subtle states of the *saṃprajñāta samādhi* without the highest *vairāgya,* are not sufficient in themselves for *asaṃprajñāta samādhi* to arise.

Sādhana: Look, listen and feel – a *bhāvana* for *saṃyama*

Although it would be a mistake to think that we can progress neatly from *dhāraṇā* to *dhyāna* and on to *samādhi*, it is possible to use *bhāvana* to deepen our involvement in a meditative practice at each of the different stages. *Dhāraṇā*, *dhyāna* and *samādhi* can be equated with looking, listening and feeling, respectively. Like all *bhāvana,* this is a creative association where the *bhāvana* evoke something of the flavour of each step (somewhat poetically). In other words, don't take these ideas too literally...

When we look at something specifically, such as a bird in a tree, we focus our eyes and watch it. We have an intention and we focus, but we are still separate. If we watch the bird intently for some time, there is a certain stability in our attention. 'Looking' as a *bhāvana* here is not limited to our visual sense. It can be linked to all our senses and means of perception. It represents the intention 'to look' in a particular direction, and to maintain the direction for some time (stability of link). It also suggests a sense of separateness (there is space between it and us). These evoke the characteristics of *dhāraṇā*.

When we really listen, we are very attentive and receptive to what is being said. 'Listening' emphasises sensitivity and receptivity, once a direction of attention has been established. Whereas 'looking' moves outwards from the subject to the object, the direction for 'listening' seems just the reverse. As a *bhāvana,* 'listening' is not restricted to our sense of hearing – an attitude beautifully summed up in the expression 'listen to your heart.' This emphasises a more sensitive and receptive state representative of *dhyāna*.

'Feeling' suggests a more immediate and sensitive contact with the object of enquiry such that it can be sensed directly. It emphasises a direct perception with no separation, as if we have become the object of meditation. Whereas we may not see clearly, or we may mishear something being said, direct feeling suggests we know something as it really *is*. This more intimate relationship evokes one of the main qualities of *samādhi*.

Spend some time '**looking**' (with all your senses), then allow yourself to consciously '**listen**' and notice the difference in the quality of your involvement. Finally, let yourself '**feel**' the object of your focus as if you have become it and can sense it directly. Spending a few minutes with each of these steps in a meditation practice, or even for a number of breaths in an āsana or prāṇāyāma with a specific focus, can lead us progressively deeper into the experience. The process is a *vinyāsa krama*, and thus needs a completion stage, so it can be useful to add a fourth stage of '**leaving**' or '**completing**' where you consciously disconnect and return to a more usual sense of awareness.

Chapter 16

ईश्वरप्रणिधानाद्वा ।

Moving Beyond Ourselves – *Īśvara* in the Yoga Sūtra

YS 1.23 īśvara praṇidhānādvā

One way to yoga is to trust in Life

Sūtra 1.23 is one of the three places in the text that reference the concept of *īśvara praṇidhāna,* which is often translated along the lines of 'surrender to the Lord' or 'devotion to God'. However, if we look at the meanings of the words, we can derive a more nuanced translation. *Īśvara* comes from the root *īś* which means 'rule' or 'command', and *vara* which implies the 'highest'. Although it is often one of the names used for the God Śiva, importantly the word is not synonymous with Śiva, or indeed any other deity. *Īśvara* is simply 'the Highest Power'; Peter Hersnack equated this with Life itself. "Life is more than each of us," he said in Montpellier in 2015. "When two people meet, there are two – but also something greater – a third. *That is Life*!"

Praṇidhāna literally means 'to bow down to', 'to revere' – and so we can understand this as 'a special attitude'. Peter translated *īśvara praṇidhāna* as 'trust in Life – with a capital L'. *Īśvara praṇidhāna* thus becomes an openness towards that which sustains us, the Life which courses through and animates all forms. To remain open to this Life is to place our trust in it. And only through placing our trust in Life, aligning ourselves with Life, can we truly be supported by it. Like our relationship with gravity, our relationship with Life can either be a battle or a support. If we are out of balance, gravity is a force we have to struggle against: if we are totally in balance, what is below will support what is above – gravity is our friend.

For most of us, a radical trust in Life is not easy; because we are out of balance we may sometimes find ourselves struggling with Life. As Patañjali repeatedly states, we must differentiate between Life and the *form that Life takes*;[1] trusting in the process and journey (i.e. Life) rather than simply being happy when things go our way and resentful when they don't (i.e. the form that Life takes). This trust comes in stages and has to be built, and it may be that we are not yet ready for this process. Importantly, the last word of sūtra 1.23, (*īśvara praṇidhānād-vā*), is *vā*. *Vā* means 'or': here Patañjali offers the practice and cultivation of a special attitude to 'the Highest' as a *possible* path to the cultivation of yoga; but if this is not something that we resonate with, he offers many other alternatives.

1. Here, Life represents *puruṣa* and the form Life takes represents *prakṛti*.

Īśvara, God, yoga and religion

At some point in their career, most yoga teachers will be asked whether yoga is a religion, whether it is part of Hinduism, and whether it requires us to believe in some form of God. Many teachers have been told that the local church hall is not a suitable place to hold classes because yoga conflicts with the particular church's (or church committee's) view of Christianity. Because many of the original teachers of yoga who brought the practice to the West in the late nineteenth and early twentieth centuries were Hindu monks,[2] there has been something of a conflation of Hinduism and yoga. Yoga in the West is sometimes adorned with Indian religious iconography – images of the various gods and goddesses as well as religious paraphernalia may not seem out of place in many yoga classes. But there are important questions here: where are the boundaries of culture, religion and spirituality? Do they intersect? How?

Desikachar was always very keen to keep the practices separate – he saw no conflict between yoga and any form of religion (or indeed, atheism). As we already said, he felt practising yoga will make a Christian a better Christian, a Muslim a better Muslim, and an atheist a better atheist. The story of his study of the Yoga Sūtra with his father (Krishnamacharya was a deeply religious man) is well known. He said that he studied the Yoga Sūtra seven times with Krishnamacharya over nearly thirty years and each time he went through the text, he was taught in a slightly different way. The first time, Desikachar asked his father to teach the sūtras with no reference to God – so he studied it as a psychological text. The last time he studied it, when Krishnamacharya was in his nineties, every sūtra was religious! Whatever Desikachar's own religious inclinations, he never adorned himself with religious markings, nor did he adopt overtly religious symbolism. He was always careful to keep his yoga teaching neutral with regard to

2. The first was Swami Vivekananda, a Vedantin monk who set up the Ramakrishna Mission.

religious sectarianism and was open to teaching all people irrespective of their religious faith (or lack of it).

Īśvara-praṇidhāna as a three-part *vinyāsa*

Throughout the text, Patañjali emphasises the process of building things slowly, carefully constructing from the ground up. This applies to all areas: body, breath, mind, and relationships. When we proceed from where we are, carefully choose a direction and take small sustainable steps in that direction, extraordinary outcomes can arise (indeed, these are the subject of Chapter 3 of the Yoga Sūtra, *Vibūhti Pāda*). When we take **support** as appropriate, allow a **direction** to reveal itself, then a new **space** manifests. This process is a dynamic interplay with each feeding the others. Krishnamacharya presented the three places where Patañjali talks of *īśvara praṇidhāna* as a *vinyāsa*; the three levels are for people at different stages of involvement or evolution in their yoga practice. The foundation level, presented at the beginning of Chapter 2 (*Sādhana Pāda*), is as a part of *kriyā yoga* (YS 2.1) – the cultivation of a stable base for one's yoga practice. In *kriyā yoga,* the priority is a reduction of problematic tendencies (that is, the *kleśa*) to a manageable level, and the cultivation of mental stability (*samādhi bhāvana*). *Kriyā yoga* is for the householder, or the beginner – someone who wants their yoga practice to support their daily life. As we have discussed, its three 'limbs' are *tapas, svādhyāya* and *īśvara praṇidhāna*. In *kriyā yoga*, the emphasis of *īśvara praṇidhāna* is more on *praṇidhāna,* the deepening and cultivation of an openness and feeling of acceptance. This feeling of acceptance is the fruit of the relationship between *tapas* and *svādhyāya*. We are disciplined (*tapas*), we cultivate self-awareness (*svādhyāya*), and this leads to a certain equanimity (*īśvara praṇidhāna*). Or, as Peter Hersnack formulated it, we take support on the external (*tapas*), we take support on the internal (*svādhyāya*), and then we take support on that which sustains both (*īśvara praṇidhāna*).

A deeper practice is presented later on in Chapter 2 (YS 2.45) as part of *aṣṭāṅga yoga* (and more specifically as part of *niyama*). Where *kriyā yoga* aims at reducing *kleśa*, *aṣṭāṅga yoga* deals with the roots of *kleśa*, not just as a palliative therapy but a radical restructuring of our hearts and minds. In this sense, we could see it as a more committed practice – for someone who wants their lifestyle to support their yoga practice. The emphasis shifts from *praṇidhāna* (attitude) towards *īśvara* (object), as we contemplate the meaning and purpose of 'Highest Power' and begin to realign our centre of gravity towards such a Power.

Just as *aparigraha* can be seen as the fruit of all the *yama*, so *īśvara praṇidhāna* can be seen as the fruit of the *niyama*. For each of the ten *yama* and *niyama*, Patañjali describes a specific fruit for when the discipline has been perfected. In YS 2.45, he states that *īśvara praṇidhāna*'s fruit is the perfection of *samādhi* (*samādhi siddhiḥ*). This is a state of mind where there is tremendous stability without rigidity; a clear and open mind allowing profound perception without our personal agenda obscuring our vision.

For someone able to sustain such *samādhi*, whose mind is stable, uncomplicated and clear, *īśvara praṇidhāna* is also presented in Chapter 1 (YS 1.23). Peter rather beautifully suggested that Chapter 1 of the Yoga Sūtra is "for one who has not lost their innocence."[3] The yogi of Chapter 1 is simple and uncluttered, and here the focus is much more on how we can understand and relate to *īśvara* (YS 1.24–28). This is akin to the path of *bhakti* – a profound and radical path to realisation, which removes our transient created identity from being centre stage of our own story.

3. Personal communication, Montpellier 2015.

Defining and relating to *īśvara*

YS 1.24 kleśa-karma-vipāka-āśayaiḥ aparāmṛṣṭaḥpuruṣa-viśeṣa īśvaraḥ

Īśvara is different to puruṣa, because there is no involvement in the karmic cycle

We can think of the essence of a person as '*puruṣa-ness*', and the essence of *puruṣa* as '*īśvara-ness*'. But just as it is a mistake to turn *puruṣa* into a 'thing' by defining it as a noun, so we must be careful in our description and conceptualisation of *īśvara. Īśvara* is here described as a special, or unique (*viśeṣa*), type of *puruṣa* – hence '*essence of puruṣa*'. But it's unhelpful to think of it as an 'it' – that would turn it into *prakṛti*! Instead, Patañjali describes *īśvara* as being free from enmeshment (*aparāmṛṣṭaḥ*) in the usual karmic cycle, and in this sense, *īśvara* can be seen as Pure Awareness, unfettered by conditioning and preconceptions. The usual pattern is a self-perpetuating merry-go-round: we act from *kleśa* which produces *karma,* this in turn bears fruit (*vipāka*) and then produces both the seed and the ground (*āśaya*) for further actions based in *kleśa*. It is a simple agricultural metaphor. *Īśvara* is free from that, because *īśvara* is free from the usual machinations of the mind – the confusions, the plotting, remembering, calculating, imagining, fearing and fantasising. *Īśvara* is simply Life itself and the actions of Life are not driven by *kleśa.*

We can understand *avidyā,* the fundamental *kleśa*, as mistaking Life for the form it takes; the latter usurps the place of the former. *Avidyā*:

- cuts us off from our relationship with Life
- creates amnesia about the precious nature of Life
- allows us to take Life for granted

Actions arising from *avidyā* invariably add to the karmic cycle, entangling us further in its knots. Life, on the other hand, doesn't suffer the karmic consequences of actions in the way we do. Although it 'acts', Life is *aparāmṛṣṭaḥ* – free from entanglement in *karma*; there is nothing for resentments, ideas and fantasies to 'stick to'.

To relate to, or indeed worship, something as abstract as 'Life', however, can be challenging. By clothing *īśvara* in names and form, we can create images to which we can aspire and align ourselves with – hence the plethora of gods in Indian religion. Each is a personification (or should we say a deification?) of some aspect or quality of Life as filtered through the human condition. The form is a conduit to help us embody certain qualities. Worship of the purely abstract is very difficult because it is elusive and intangible. For developing fearlessness, a devotee might worship the monkey god, Hanuman. For cultivating intellect or musicianship, another may worship the goddess Saraswati. A follower of Christ may hope to enkindle feelings of compassion. To worship the principle of destruction (and renewal), Śiva and Kāli are both honoured. However, any of these paths can lead to sectarianism, whereby the *praṇidhāna* simply becomes the worship of empty idols: a confusion of the map with the territory. A helpful image of *īśvara* should point us to something which is greater than each one of us (and indeed, greater than any single image of divinity), ever present and unfettered by mental noise.

YS 1.25 tatra niratiśayaṃ sarva-jñabījam

There is the unsurpassed seed of all wisdom

How do we learn? Where does knowledge come from? All sacred teachings were divided into two categories in Ancient India: *śruti* (revealed or heard) and *smṛti* (remembered). For the Ancients, only the Veda were truly *śruti*. They were understood to be divinely inspired, intuited from beyond the worldly realm. All texts which are not *śruti* are *smṛti*, arising from observation or reasoning and passed on by tradition. However brilliant, they are not seen as divinely inspired. The Yoga Sūtra, for example, is a *smṛti* text, but by seeing Patañjali as part of a long tradition (*anuśāsanam*) and viewing the text as aligned with the Veda, there is a suggestion of the inspiration for the text originating, or deriving from, divine intuition.

In order to gain wisdom (*jñā*), we need to be able to perceive well. The three means of knowing as described by Patañjali (YS 1.6) are direct perception (*pratyakṣa*), inference (*anumāna*) and received wisdom (*āgama*). These three often form a *vinyāsa*: first we are told (*āgama*), then we infer (*anumāna*) and finally we see directly (*pratyakṣa*).[4] But even behind that, behind being told – what is the seed (*bīja*) of knowledge?

Īśvara is described as a 'special type of *puruṣa*' (*puruṣa-viśeṣa*), one who sees without distortion or projection. *Īśvara* is thus a model of clear perception for us to draw inspiration from and aspire to. We can begin to align ourselves with this ideal. Through the process of yoga, direct perception (*pratyakṣa*) produces wisdom (*jñāna*) and we perceive something of Life itself. A new and direct perception dawns, revealing that which connects everything, the inter-relationship of all becomes clear. This is called *yaugika pratyakṣa* – the direct perception of Life unfettered by inference or Tradition. It is, in a sense, the perception of *īśvara*.

YS 1.26 sa eṣa pūrveṣāmapi guruḥ kālenānavacchedāt

In this way, because it has no limits, it is the Teacher of all previous teachers

The term 'guru' can be poetically derived by breaking it into two syllables – '*gu*' means dark and '*ru*' is light. Thus a *guru* is 'one who brings light to where there is darkness'. Passing teachings on is not about one person giving the next generation the antique family heirloom, but rather about the light from one igniting the light in the next. This makes it alive; the teachings are not based in the past and confined

4. There are exceptions to this. In the *Sāṃkhya Kārikā*, Īśvara Kṛṣṇa says that there are a number of reasons that an object can never be seen directly (e.g. it is too subtle or too big). In such cases we need to use inference or testimony.

by time (*kālenānavacchedāt*). Instead, they are limitless; like the very present moment, they are always fresh. Now is the perfect moment to wake up, so don't worry – we don't simply 'miss the moment' for it never to be repeated! All previous teachers (*pūrveṣāmapi guruḥ*) have 'come alight' in the present moment by their direct perception of Life itself – and the role of the teacher is to help ignite the flame already waiting to be lit in each one of us.

YS 1.27 tasya vācakaḥ praṇavaḥ

Sacred sounds are the means to connect

Although one of the common symptoms of mental illness is hearing voices, actually most of us have a near continuous stream of words and voices running through our minds for much of the time. Not only that, but often these voices can be punitive or negative and by their (usually unconscious) repetition, our lives and views of ourselves and the world we live in are shaped. This is exactly why mantra is said to be such an important practice; it is a tool for reshaping our minds and therefore our reality. Just as āsana and prāṇāyāma can be used in different ways – as a therapy, for empowerment, or to prepare for meditative practices – so too can mantra. This is the *viniyoga* of mantra. There are mantras for gaining wealth, for healing and even for cursing. Here in the Yoga Sūtra, the purpose is very specific: to open a channel to the Transcendent and thereby reshape our identity.

In Sanskrit, the naming of something – *nāma* – is extremely important because it helps to colour our understanding of events and objects. By becoming the symbol for something, naming 'clothes' naked experience. The voicing of that symbol, whether performed aloud or silently, is *vācaka*.

Patañjali is very careful not to use any specific term for *īśvara*; instead, he says that the way to relate to *īśvara* is through the voicing of *praṇava*. In conventional understanding, *praṇava* means the symbol Oṃ, and this is certainly true for Hindus. However, Desikachar was insistent that we should not confuse the two: for a Hindu *praṇava* may be Oṃ, but for others, a different symbol or sound can be equally sacred and an appropriate medium for a relationship with the Transcendent. There are, however, specific qualities of the sound Oṃ which *do* make it very special – it is said to encompass all sounds because its first sound is *a* and it finishes with *ṃ* – the last sound in Sanskrit. Thus everything that can be spoken (from *a* to *ṃ*) is contained within the sound. There is an interesting convention that states that there is always a brief silence after vocalising Oṃ, and this silence represents all that cannot be expressed in words or concepts. In this way, Oṃ plus the silence encompasses everything – that which can be expressed (*prakṛti*) and that which cannot (*puruṣa* and *īśvara*).

ॐ

The symbol 'Oṃ'

YS 1.28 taj-japaḥ tad-artha-bhāvanam

Repetition (of praṇava) should be accompanied by meditation on its purpose and meaning

We have seen how in *dhāraṇā,* there is a constant practice of returning the mind to an object of focus. Through this process, *dhāraṇā* develops into *dhyāna,* and finally into *samādhi*. Even here, in *samādhi,* there are increasing levels of subtlety with correspondingly rarefied thoughts, feelings and ideas. Akin to this process is the practice of *japa,* which Patañjali here states is the way of coming into relationship with *īśvara*. *Japa* is the repetition of a sacred word or mantra; often beads threaded on a cord are used to count the number of repetitions (these beads are called *mālā*).

When we use mantra or *japa*, there is also a hierarchy

to the vocalisation. Initially, we chant out loud; this is the grossest level because it is most tangible and audible. This is called *vācika* ('voiced'). To make the practice more silent and also more internal, the next level is one of 'mouthing' – we produce the shapes of the words with our vocal apparatus, but there is hardly any sound, just the faint whisper of the breath. This is called *upāṃṣu*. And finally there is silent repetition, where the sound is purely mental (*mānasa*). This is seen as the most subtle practice of *japa*. Each practice is a deepening of the previous level and our involvement becomes more internal.

However, mindlessly repeating a mantra is not enough. There needs to be some consideration of what the mantra is pointing towards, lest we spend all of our time simply engaging with a symbol. The symbol is a pointer; that is its purpose (*artha*) and if we get stuck on the symbol, we may find ourselves 'eating the menu'. The symbol points us to 'the Highest' and its purpose is to move us closer to Life itself – to trust in and be supported by Life's currents. It is sometimes difficult to surrender to these currents, to trust in their direction and to allow ourselves to be carried. However, this trust is a process of alignment with Life, allowing a new consciousness to 'come into being' (*bhāvana*) and for Patañjali, the primary technique for this alignment is *japa*.

Sādhana: *Bhāvana* and being carried

Bhāvana

One of the iconic images of Walt Disney's 1961 feature film *One Hundred and One Dalmatians* is of dog owners walking their particular pets with an uncanny (and very amusing) mirroring between humans and animals. It is a well-known cliché that dogs begin to resemble their owners (or is it the other way round?). Certainly one of the premises of yoga psychology is that we become what we think – the more we focus on something, the more it colours our minds and creates a reality. For many, the ultimate ascetic is the dreadlocked Śiva. For others, Christ is a symbol of loving kindness and compassion, and for others still Buddha's steadiness and wisdom make him an inspiration as they move towards cultivating these qualities within themselves. Focusing on the attributes of any of these luminaries slowly changes the qualities of our minds; it is a simple and pragmatic idea.

It's interesting that Patañjali uses the term *bhāvana* in YS 1.28. Although we often use the word in the context of āsana or prāṇāyāma practice to indicate an image, or a visualisation which can help to establish the form of a posture or enrich a technique, it's important to not think of *bhāvana* as just a flavouring – something which we add to the main body of a posture to bring out a particular aspect. This potentially trivialises a concept and practice at the very heart of the yoga project: *bhāvana* is an essential element of *sādhana*.

The word is derived from the root *bhū* meaning 'to be'. The suffix '*–ana*' means 'an instrument of' (there are lots of Sanskrit words that end with this suffix, and understanding this will help to make sense of their meaning). So we could say that *bhāvana* is literally 'an instrument of becoming': it allows something to come into being. Often in āsana and prāṇāyāma, a *bhāvana* is more ambiguous than a simple instruction – there is room for play and imagination. This is important: it is an invitation to creatively engage with the imagery of *bhāvana* and discover something of our own feelings and our own sense of Being. To focus on the qualities of a particular deity as a *bhāvana* helps us to cultivate those very qualities within ourselves.

We have seen how Patañjali's primary tool for *īśvara praṇidhāna* is *japa*, the repetition and contemplation of sacred sounds. As we have already suggested, āsana can be seen as the 'poetry of the body'. Although a modern idea, we can also think of the repetition of certain movements and bodily shapes, and the conscious control of the breath, as a form of *japa* – that is, a way of cultivating a new awareness and sense of being, through repetition.

In āsana, *bhāvana* help us to inhabit a posture in a special way and thus have a particular experience of the posture. Sometimes the very name of a posture can be a *bhāvana*: cobra (*bhujaṅgāsana)*, warrior (*vīrabhadrāsana*), mountain (*tāḍāsana*). When we think of a cobra's hood, it allows our chest to expand laterally as we come into *bhujaṅgāsana*. The warrior is both a great force of nature, but also a servant – so although when we practise *vīrabhadrāsana* we have vigour and power, it can be tempered by a certain feeling of humility. A mountain is stable, noble, dignified and tall. These images can certainly inform our practice of *tāḍāsana*. Sometimes a *bhāvana* can involve placing the attention in a particular area: 'root the feet' or 'open the flank'. *Bhāvana* can also convey a way of performing an action: 'let the arms float', 'let the body fly', 'let the pelvis drop'.

In prāṇāyāma, *bhāvana* can help us to feel deeply engaged with subtle energies that are manipulated by our very breath. One of the functions of *prāṇa vāyu* is to connect and create passageways for communication, and it is chiefly influenced by our in-breath. Thus we may feel the inhalation 'opening the axis' or 'linking the nostril to the heart'. We may even feel it 'igniting our form'. Similarly, our out-breath is said to influence *apāna vāyu*. We may feel the exhalation 'ungluing itself from the form', 'withdrawing from the pelvis' and yet 'maintaining space and not collapsing the form'.

Bhāvana are always a mixture of the imaginary and the real; they require us to engage our attention and imagination, but there needs to be some sort of logic or truth in the imagery. With skilful and intelligent use, we can often be surprised and delighted by the responses of our bodies and breath when we use *bhāvana*. Most importantly, they are pointers inviting us to experience something beyond ourselves; they function as portals to a new way of being. We are touched and reshaped by the experience of *bhāvana*.

Whilst there are many *bhāvana* to help us experience subtle energies or feelings within the practice of both āsana and prāṇāyāma, the most important is to feel the body as light, spacious, and also a vehicle for Life to dance within. Our bodies are sacred spaces which allow Life expression; our breath is the evidence of that very expression.

Being carried

We have already seen how the concept of taking support requires that we do just that – allow ourselves to be held by support. For many people growing up in our contemporary Western culture, there is an insidious feeling of 'unworthiness' – at a deep level many feel they are neither deserving, nor essentially beautiful. It is interesting to contrast this deep under-confidence with the feeling of entitlement – for example, the promotion of rights. We deserve this or that (often a luxury); or we don't deserve something (how can we say whether or not some suffering is 'deserved' or not?). Perhaps the myth of 'original sin' has left us in a place where we feel that our essence is polluted and that we must do all we can to purify this very essence; while simultaneously feeling indignation when reality deviates from our desires. As we have seen, traditional Indian thought does not see our very essence as polluted, or in need of therapeutic interventions. Underneath the covering, the conditioning and confusion, yoga proposes that we are perfect; but this requires us to understand that we are indeed held by Life itself.

One way that we can consciously practise this feeling of being supported is in *śavāsana*. Although it is not a posture that was taught a great deal by Krishnamacharya (other than as a brief rest to recover from a strenuous series of āsana), it does offer some very interesting possibilities for conscious practice. The danger of *śavāsana* is that as *rajas* reduces, the mind has two options – either to slip into *tamas* or become illumined by *sattva*. If we stay too long in *śavāsana,* we may simply go to sleep – *tamas* predominates and we fall into slumber. Perhaps that is what was needed – but it is not really yoga where the goal is the cultivation of *sattva*. A very effective *bhāvana* to use in *śavāsana* is to trust in your support, knowing you will be held. Sometimes we use the idea that the more we can allow ourselves to be carried by the earth below us, the more we can open to the sky above us. Many people are profoundly affected by this simple suggestion; it gives permission to let go of something very deeply and open to new possibilities without fear. In this sense, it allows us to move beyond ourselves and trust in Life.

Glossary

Notes on Sanskrit

Diacritics

The most common script for writing Sanskrit or Hindi in modern India is *devanāgarī*. It is a common misconception that Sanskrit (*ṣaṃskṛta*) **is** *devanāgarī*; in fact, Sanskrit has been written in many different scripts over its long history, and indeed was originally an oral language with no written form. Thus, Sanskrit may be represented in the Roman script in different ways and a number of 'standard' transliteration systems have evolved.

We have adopted the IAST (International Alphabet of Sanskrit Transliteration) system which uses a series of diacritic marks to represent the range of Sanskrit characters (there are more characters in Sanskrit than in English). Although not a phonetic representation of Sanskrit, it has the advantage of representing each Sanskrit character uniquely, which many of the phonetic systems without diacritics do not.

Pronunciation

There are many books and resources available that provide a pronunciation guide to Sanskrit and so we have chosen not to go into too much detail. However, a few well-chosen remarks will help to guide the reader in avoiding the most obvious errors. In our experience, the single most important thing that a native English speaker can do to make words sound roughly correct is to pronounce the vowels correctly and differentiate between 'short' and 'long' vowels. Long vowels are given twice as much 'air time' as short vowels, and are generally emphasised. The short vowels are *a, i, u* and *ṛ*, and the long vowels are ā, ī, ū, e, o, *ai* and *au* (although *ai* and *au* are two letters, they represent single Sanskrit vowels). Making the short vowels short, and the long vowels long is key!

Native English speakers naturally emphasise the penultimate syllable of a word. For example, mispronouncing āsana as 'as<u>aa</u>na', as opposed to the correct '<u>aa</u>sunu' (the two short *a*-es like the 'u' in 'sun'). Similarly, first and last 'a's in *dhāraṇā* are elongated.

Sanskrit roots: The source of everything

In ancient times the oral language of Sanskrit was analysed by Indian grammarians and organised into a formal structure. This was a monumentally complex task requiring the shoe-horning of the language into some kind of system. This system then became a benchmark for the Sanskrit that followed, particularly with regard to erudite philosophical texts. According to grammatical tradition, all Sanskrit words come from a set of approximately 2,000 verbal roots (*dhātu*) which are then used to form nouns and verbs according to various rules. It is common to understand words and make links between words by analysing their roots. For example, the root of the word āsana is *ās* – to sit.

Why are there so many different forms of the same word?

Sanskrit is an inflected language: the form of a word changes to express grammatical function such as tense, mood, person or case. Typically the endings of words change, so as a subject of a sentence we might have one *āsanam* (posture) and many *āsanāni* (postures). With nouns there is also a theoretical stem form to which the endings are added and this is generally what we use when explaining a Sanskrit noun in isolation. Hence, we explain the meaning of the word āsana (stem form) which appears in YS 2.47 as *sthira sukham āsanam* (where the grammatical ending has been added).

The situation becomes a little more complex with the principle of *sandhi* (joining together). In Sanskrit, the often subtle changes in pronunciation that occur when two words are pronounced sequentially are reflected in the written language: typically the ending of the first word changes and the two words may join together. So for example '*tat artha*' becomes *tadartha*. Or the familiar phrase *śāntiḥ śāntiḥ śāntiḥ* is written '*śāntiṣṣāntiśśantiḥ*'.

We are not suggesting that yoga students need to become Sanskrit scholars, but understanding some rules about how the language works can help you to recognise the more common forms.

Sanskrit compounds

Compounds are nouns linked together with the relationship between them understood but not explicitly stated (in English we often express relationships between words explicitly with prepositions and conjunctions, such as 'of', 'by' and 'and'). There are a number of types of compounds in Sanskrit. The Yoga Sūtra is full of compounds and this is the source of many differences of translation and interpretation. In YS 2.47, for example, *sthirasukham* is a compound of the words *sthira* and *sukha*. The relationship between them is inferred and understood in this context as indicating that that āsana is defined by the qualities of *sthira* **and** *sukha*. But theoretically it could be different: *sukha* may be achieved **by means of** *sthira*.

Glossary

We have listed the Sanskrit terms in an English alphabetical order as though all the letters were English and without diacritics. Strictly speaking this is a nonsense, because it ignores the significance of the different Sanskrit letters, but from a practical point of view, it is much easier for English speakers to quickly find the word and its definition.

Glossary of Sanskrit terms

abhāva – not arising, not becoming
abhibhava – overpowering
abhimata – agreeable, desired
abhiniveśa – profound fear (ultimately, of death); clinging to life
abhyantara – the 'inner' domain
abhyantara vṛtti – the movement towards the inside i.e. the inhale
abhyāsa – diligent practice, the effort to stay with something
ādara – enthusiasm, zeal
ādaya – and the rest, etc., from *ādi*
ādhibhautika duḥkha – suffering caused by other creatures
ādhidaivika duḥkha – suffering caused by divine forces
adhikāra – qualification or suitability for something
adhimātra – intense
adho mukha – downward facing
ādhyātmika duḥkh – suffering caused by myself
adhyāya – chapter or section
adhyayana – Vedic chanting, study
agni – fire (often related to our health and vitality when used in certain contexts)
āhāra – food
ahiṃsā – non-violence
ajñāna – misunderstanding
ākāśa – the 'element' of space
ākṣepī – transcended
alabdhabhūmikatva – failing to actualise or to reach a goal
ālambana – support, something to rest on
ālasya – dullness, lack of lustre
āma – undigested material
amṛta – elixir of immortality
anāgata – in the future, yet to come
anavasthitatvāni – slipping back, instability
ānanda – bliss, joy
ananta – mythical serpent, also 'without end' or infinite
anātma – not-self, non-essential
anavaccheda – unseparated, unlimited, unbounded
anavacchinna – unlimited, unbounded
aṅga – limb
aṅgamejayatva – trembling of the limbs (and by implication, body instability)
anitya – impermanent
antarāya – obstacle or interruption
antaraṅga – inner limbs, usually with reference to the last three of Patañjali's eight limbs
antar kumbhaka – the pause at the end of the inhale (AK); literally 'holding within' (*antar*)
anugama – following on from
anukāra – resembling
anuloma – with the hair, with the grain
anuloma ujjāyī – *prāṇāyāma* technique in which the exhale is directed through alternate nostrils; literally 'with-the-hair *ujjāyī*'
anumodita – approved, agreeable
anuśāsana – a wisdom teaching (to be followed and practised)
anuśayī – flowing on from
ānuśravika – 'that which has been heard', referring to spiritual aspirations and goals
anuttama – unsurpassed
anya – other
apāna – the energetic principle associated with elimination, often described as *apāna vāyu*
aparāmṛṣṭa – untouched, free from, untainted
aparigraha – non grasping
āpatti – falling into, entering a state or condition
apavarga – freedom, liberation
aprīti – pain
artha – purpose or essence
āsana – originally a seat, or seated posture; later it came to mean any yoga posture
āśaya – deposit, residue
asaṃprayoga – disconnection, separation
asaṃprajñāta – not accompanied by wisdom or insight
asaṃsarga – lack of contact
āsevita – cultivated, practised diligently
asmitā – the sense of self, literally 'I-am-ness'
āśrama – stage of life
āśraya – support
āśrayatva – connectness, correspondence with
aṣṭāṅga – eight-limbed
asura – demon
aśuci – impure
aśuddhi – impurity
asteya – not stealing
atha – now
ātmaka – nature, belonging to
ātman – Self, essence
āvaraṇa – that which obscures (synonymous with *tamas*)
avasthāna – dwelling, abiding, standing
avidyā – misunderstanding
avirati – intemperance, over-indulgence
āyāma – stretching, extending
āyurveda – traditional Indian medical system

bādhana – bondage, oppression
bahir aṅga – external limbs, usually with reference to the first five of Patañjali's eight limbs
bāhya kumbhaka – holding outside *(bāhya)*, the pause at the end of the exhale
bāhya vṛtti – the movement towards the outside i.e. the exhale
bandha – lock or seal
Bhagavad Gītā – song (*gītā*) of the Lord (*bhagavan*)
Bhagīratha – name of legendary sage
Bṛhadāraṇyaka Upaniṣad – the 'Great Forest' *upaniṣad*
bhakti – devotion
bhastrikā – prāṇāyāma technique that combines rapid breathing and nostril control, literally 'bellows'
bhauma – occasion, circumstance
bhāvana – feeling, cultivation of something, means to bring something into being
bhoga – experience, enjoyment
bhrāmarī – *prāṇāyāma* technique that involves humming like a bee, literally 'relating to a bee'
bhrāntidarśana – confusion, wrong view
bhūmi – level, ground, situation
bhūta – element, being
brahmacarya – discipline, or as one of the four stages of life, studentship
brahma/brahman – the absolute
Brahma – the creator God, one of the trinity that includes Viṣṇu and Śiva
brahmavihāra – the disposition or abode of Brahma
bṛṃhaṇa – expanding
buddhi – the most subtle part of the mind
cakravāka – mythical bird
cala – moving
candra – the moon
caturtha – the fourth
cetanā – consciousness, state of mind
cikitsā – healing practice, therapy
cit – 'pure awareness' or 'true self' (synonymous with *puruṣa*)
citta – the mind 'that which relates to or is subservient to *cit*'
darśana – point of view, often used as designating a philosophical view
daurmanasya – negative thinking, pessimism, literally 'bad mind'
deśa – place
deva – god, a class of divine beings
devaloka – realm of the gods
devatā – form of God or the divine
dhāraṇā – holding the mind to a point of focus
dharma – our responsibilities and purpose in life, the order of things, fundamental nature
dhyāna – contemplation, meditation
dīrgha – long (of the breath)
dīrghakāla – a long time
doṣa – fault, defect
draṣṭṛ – 'the one who sees' (synonymous with *puruṣa* or *cit*)
dṛḍhabhūmi – stability, solid ground, firmly established
dṛś – the seer, one who sees (appears as *dṛk/dṛg*)
dṛṣṭa – what is seen, material objects
dṛśya – the observable world, the 'seen' (synonymous with *prakṛti*)
duḥkha – limited or restricted space, usually translated as pain, suffering or distress
dveṣa – habitual aversion
dvandva – pairs
eka – one
ekāgrya – one-pointedness
ekāgra – one-pointed
ekatānatā – single continuity
eka tattva – a single or essential principle
ekātmatā – a single entity, a single continuity
ekatra – in one place, together
Gaṅgā – the goddess personifying the river Ganges
gati – movement or flow
graha – grasped
gṛhastha – householder
gomukha – cow face
guṇa – literally quality, often referring to the *triguṇa* of *rajas*, *tamas* and *sattva*
guru – teacher, literally heavy
hāna – that which is to be given up or relinquished
haṭha – 'forceful', symbolically understood as 'sun and moon'
hetu – cause
heya – that which is to be overcome or avoided
hiṃsā – violence
iḍā – *nāḍī* originating at left nostril
indriya – senses/the organs of our senses
iṣṭa – chosen, desired
īśvara – a higher power, the Lord, God
Īśvara Kṛṣṇa – author of *Sāṃkhya Kārika*
itaratra – at other times, elsewhere
iva – as if
jala – water
jālandhara – 'water holder' as in *jālandhara bandha*
janana – generating, giving birth to
janma – birth, circumstances of life

japa – meditation using repetition of a mantra
jāti – birth
jñāna – knowledge
jugupsā – dislike, disgust
jyotiṣmatī – having light, luminous
kaivalya – freedom, literally 'aloneness'
kāla – time
kāma – sensual pleasure and enjoyment
kapālabhāti – a *krīya* (cleansing action) involving rapid breathing controlled using the abdominal muscles, literally 'shining skull'
kārita – caused
karma – action
katham – how
kathaṃtā – 'how-ness', the nature of something
Kaṭha Upaniṣad – the *upaniṣad* of the sage Kaṭha
kāya – body
khecarī – a Haṭha yoga practice that involves turning the tongue backwards in the mouth
khyāti – perception, knowledge
kleśa – an affliction, something that will cause distress
karuṇā – compassion
kriyā – activity, action, in the Yoga Sūtra used as a name for *rajas*
kṣaya – destruction, reduction
kṣipta – scattered, deranged
kṣiyate – dissolved, diminished
kṣema – well-founded, secure or maintained
krodha – anger
kṛta – deed, or action that has been done
kṣetra – field, ground
kumbhaka – pot or vessel
lābha – obtaining, attaining
lakṣaṇa – essential quality, mark, sign
laya krama – the phase of dissolution, old age
laghu – light
laṅghana – making light, fasting
lobha – greed
madhya – moderate, middling
Mahābhārata – epic narrative, the 'great tale of the Bharat dynasty'
mahāvrata – great vow or commitment
maitrī – friendliness
mālā – garland, rosary
manas – the mind, particularly the coordinating and thinking aspect of the mind
mānasa – mental, of the mind
mantra – a word or phrase that is repeated in meditation, literally 'instrument of the mind'
mātra – only, exclusively
miśra – mixed
mithuna – pairing, copulation
moha – delusion
mokṣa – liberation
mṛgi mudrā – hand position used to control the breath in the nostrils during prāṇāyāma, literally 'the symbol of a deer'
mṛdu – mild, weak
muditā – goodwill, joy, gladness
mudrā – a seal or gesture
mūla – the root
mūrchā – prāṇāyāma technique in which the exhale is lengthened to the maximum, literally 'swoon or faint'
nāḍī śodhana – prāṇāyāma technique in which the breath is directed through alternate nostrils, literally 'purification of the channels (*nāḍī*)'
nāḍī – river or channel
nairantarya – without interruption
nāma – name
Narasimha – an incarnation of *viṣṇu*, half-man and half-lion
niratiśaya – unsurpassed
Naṭarāja – Lord of the Dance, Śiva
nidrā – dreamless sleep
nirbhāsa – shining out, appearance
nirbīja – without seed
nirguṇa – without qualities
nirodha – a state of arrest, restraint, obstruction, covering
niruddha – alternative term for the state of *nirodha*
nitya – permanent
niyama – restraint, personal discipline
niyoga – application
nyāsa – placing, applying
ojas – vigour, the most refined product of the digestive process according to āyurveda
Oṃ – sacred syllable
pāda – foot, root, verse or chapter
pañca – five
paramparā – 'from one to another', lineage or the sequence of transmission in a tradition
para – other
paridṛṣṭa – viewed from all around
pariṇāma – the process of change
paripāka – cooked on all sides
parivṛtti – twisting, turning around
pārśva – flank, side
pat – to fall
phala – fruit
piṅgalā – *nāḍī* originating at right nostril
plāvinī – prāṇāyāma technique involving a long hold after inhalation, literally 'that which causes floating'
Prajāpati – the primordial person, literally 'the Lord of creatures'
prakāśa – luminosity, 'that which shines', in the Yoga Sūtra used as a name for sattva

prakṛti – the phenomenal world, everything of which we can be aware, also our natural constitutional state in āyurveda
pramāda – intoxication or obsession
prāṇa – life force or energy, literally that which 'travels well', connected with the breath
prāṇacalana – circulation of energy
prāṇāyāma – seated breathing practice, literally: the concentration of vital energy
prāṇasthāna – the place of *prāṇa* (i.e. the chest)
praṇava – sacred sound or symbol, traditionally taken as Oṃ
praṇidhāna – surrender, devotion, literally 'placing down in front of'
prasādana – clear, peaceful, calm
praśānta vāhitā – a peaceful flow
prasupta – dormant
praśvāsa – breathing out
pratikriyā – opposite action
pratikriyāsana – opposite action posture, counter-posture
pratiloma ujjāyī – a prāṇāyāma technique using a combination of *anuloma ujjāyī* and *viloma ujjāyī*
pratipakṣa – the other 'wing', the other side, alternative view
pratiprasava – against the flow, returning to the origin
pratiṣṭhā – established, grounded
pratyakcetanā – inward-looking consciousness
pratyāhāra – withdrawal of the senses
prayatna – special effort
pratyaya – idea, response in mind to a perception
pravṛtti – activity towards, appearance
prīti – joy
puṇya – virtuous, auspicious
pura – a city or palace
pūraka – filling up, inhaling
puruṣa – 'dweller in the city,' the essence of a person, pure awareness
puruṣārtha – the aims or purpose of life
pūrva – former, earlier, preceding
pūrvaka – preceding
pūrvāṅga – preliminary limbs, preparation
rāga – habitual desire
rahasya – secret
rajas – one of the *triguṇa*, literally 'that which colours', associated with activity and stimulation
rakṣaṇa – protective, as in *rakṣaṇa krama*; a protective or maintenance practice
ratna – jewel
recaka – emptying, exhalation
ṛṣi – sage or seer
ṛta – eternal truth, divine law
rudh – root of *nirodha*, meaning to obstruct, arrest, restrain or cover
rūpa – form, appearance
sabīja – with seed
sādhana – the means to achieve something, the practices that one adopts
saguṇa – with qualities
śaithilya – relaxation, making loose or smooth
śakti – energy, power
samādhi – a deep state of complete meditative absorption
śamana – calming, soothing
samantraka – with mantra, usually with reference to prāṇāyāma accompanied by mental recitation of word or phrase
samāpatti – a state of meditative absorption, to join or 'fall into' completely
samārūdha – firmly rooted
samavṛtti – equal movements or equal parts
samaya – circumstance, condition
sannidhi – nearness, proximity
saṃkhyā – number
saṃnyāsin – renunciate
saṃprajñāta – accompanied by wisdom
saṃprayoga – contact with
saṃśaya – doubt
saṃskāra – habit, impression in the mind that causes habitual pattern of thought or action
saṃtoṣa – contentment
saṃyama – meditative enquiry, literally 'completely restraining or holding'
saṃyoga – complete linking, in the Yoga Sūtra used in a negative context to suggest a confused relationship
śaṇmukhī – the whole face, as in *śaṇmukhī mudrā*
sārūpya – similarity of form
sarva – all
sārva – universal, another grammatical form of *sarva*
sat – true, right, real, 'being'
satkāra – 'doing it right', doing something with care
satsaṅga – good company, good association
sattva – one of the *triguṇa*, literally pure being, associated with clarity and lightness
satya – truthfulness
saumanasya – cheerfulness, positivity
śauca – cleansing, purity, cleanliness, 'that which shines'
śeṣa – remainder, residue
siddhi – power, mastery, accomplishment
śikṣaṇa – teaching, as in *śikṣaṇa krama*; an

uncompromised or classical practice
śīla – nature, disposition
śītalī – a prāṇāyāma technique in which one breathes in through the curled tongue extended beyond the lips, literally 'cooling'
sītkārī – a prāṇāyāma technique in which one breathes in through the mouth, literally 'making the sound *sīt*'
Śiva – literally 'the auspicious one', the God of destruction and transformation
smita – smiling, smile
śodhana – cleansing
sṛṣṭi krama – the phase of growth, youth
śraddhā – faith, trust, conviction, literally 'holding to truth'
śruti – 'that which has been heard', referring to texts said to be of divine origin
stambha vṛtti – a suspended movement, the pause between inhale and exhale, or between exhale and inhale
sthira – firmness, stability
sthairya – stability (having the quality of *sthira*)
sthiti – standing, remaining, stability, in the Yoga Sūtra used as a name for *tamas*
sthiti krama – the phase of stability, middle age
styāna – stagnation, rigidity
śuci – pure
śuddhi – purity
sukha – ease, 'free space', comfort, happiness, bliss
sūkṣma – subtle
śūnya – empty
sūrya bhedana – a prāṇāyāma technique in which inhalation is directed through the right nostril and exhalation through the left nostril, literally 'piercing the sun'
sva – self, one's own
svādhyāya – reciting or studying sacred texts, repetition of mantra, literally 'moving towards the Self'
svāṅga – 'one's own limbs'
śvāsapraśvāsa – literally 'inhale-exhale', but understood in āyurveda and the Yoga Sūtra as a disturbed, irregular or unconscious breathing pattern
svarasa – taste of oneself
śvāsa – breathing in
svastha – 'established in oneself', the term for health in āyurveda
svapna – dream
tad – that
tamas – one of the *triguṇa*, literally 'darkness', associated with heaviness and obscuration
tanu – thin, small
tāpa – pain, heat, anguish
tapas – heat, discipline, setting and observing boundaries
tapasvin – one who engages in *tapas*
tasminsati – established in this
tatas – there, then, usually appears as *tataḥ*
tattva – essential principle, literally 'that-ness'
traya – a 'three', triplet
tyāga – giving up, abandoning
udāra – fully arisen
ujjāyī – literally 'mastery of the upward', a means of regulating the flow of the breath
upāṃśu – at the lips
upāya – means, method
upastambhaka – exciting, stimulating
upasthāna – coming near, presence
upekṣa – equanimity
utpanna – arisen, produced
vā – 'or', in some cases, 'and'
vācaka – sound, verbal expression
vācika – voiced
vāhi – carrying or bearing
vairāgya – detachment, openness
vaira – hostility
vanaprastha – 'forest dweller', the third of the Vedic life stages
varaṇaka – obscuring, covering
vaśīkāra – complete mastery
vāyu – wind, often a synonym for *prāṇa*
vibhūti – 'special powers', the name of the third chapter of Yoga Sūtra
vicāra – contemplation, in Yoga Sūtra indicates a subtle level of perception
vicchinna – interrupted, cut off before their prime
viccheda – cutting or regulating
viduṣa – wise one, sage
vidyā – knowing, knowledge
vijñāna – wisdom
vikṛti – a state of imbalance, away from our *prakṛti*
viloma – against the hair, against the grain
viloma ujjāyī – prāṇāyāma technique in which the inhale is directed through alternate nostrils, literally 'against-the-hair *ujjāyī*'
viniyoga – special or specific application (from *viśeṣa* – special or specific, and *niyoga* – application)
vinyāsa – an arrangement or placing in a particular way
vinyāsa krama – a special or intelligent arrangement to progress in steps

vipāka – fruit, effect, result
virāma – cessation
vīrya – vitality, vigour, strength
viṣāda – despair
viṣamavṛtti – unequal movements or unequal parts
viṣaya – object of sensory perception
viśeṣa – special or specific
Viṣṇu – the God who preserves or sustains, one of the trinity that includes Brahma and Śiva
viśokā – without sorrow
vīta – free, released
vitarka – conceptual or discursive thought
viveka – discrimination or discernment
vrata – vow or commitment
vṛddhi – growth
vṛtti – a 'turning', movement, activity
vyādhi – sickness, literally 'displaced'
vyutthāna – emergence, arising
yama – restraint or attitude
yatna – effort
yogyatva – fitness or suitability for
yogyatā – fitness or suitability for
yatna – effort

Āsana glossary

adho mukha śvānāsana – downward facing dog posture
apānāsana – knee-to-chest posture
ardha matsyendrāsana – seated twist, literally 'the half-posture of Matsyendra'
bhagīrathāsana – posture of sage Bhagīratha (also known as *vṛkṣāsana*, or tree posture)
bhujaṅgāsana – cobra posture
cakravākāsana – cat posture (although *cakravāka* is in fact a mythical bird)
daṇḍāsana – staff posture
dhanurāsana – bow posture
dvi pāda pīṭham – two foot support
gomukhāsana – cow's face posture
halāsana – plough posture
jānuśīrṣāsana – head-to-knee posture
jaṭhara parivṛtti – lying twist, literally 'churning of the abdomen'
kapotāsana – pigeon posture
kūrmāsana – turtle posture
mahā mudrā – the great seal
padmāsana – lotus posture
pārśva uttānāsana – flank forward bend
paścimatānāsana – symmetrical seated forward bend, literally 'west side' stretch posture
śalabhāsana – locust posture
samasthiti – equally or evenly stable, standing with attention
sarvāṅgāsana – shoulderstand, literally 'all limbs posture'
śavāsana – corpse posture
śīrṣāsana – headstand
siṃhāsana – lion posture
tāḍāsana – mountain posture
trikonāsana – triangle posture
ūrdhva dhanurāsana – elevated or upward bow posture (often known as 'the wheel')
utkaṭāsana – squat, literally 'fierce' posture
uttānāsana – standing forward bend, literally intense stretch posture
vajrāsana – kneeling posture
vīrabhadrāsana – warrior posture (Vīrabhadra was a mythical hero)

Bibliography

Yoga Sūtra

Bharati, Swami Veda. 2015. *Yoga Sūtras of Patañjali Volume 1 Samādi-Pāda*. New Delhi: Motilal Banarsidass.
An extensive and thorough translation (including Vyāsa's commentary) of Chapter 1 of the Yoga Sūtra.

Bouanchaud, Bernard. 1997. *The Essence of Yoga*. Oregon: Portland Press.
A translation and commentary by one of Desikachar's senior students. Translated from French – which can make it slightly clumsy in places.

Bryant, Edwin. 2009. *The Yoga Sūtras of Patañjali*. New York: North Point Press.
Academic but approachable. Includes a word-for-word translation, with extensive material from the major traditional commentators.

Chapple, Christopher. 1990. *The Yoga Sūtras of Patañjali*. Delhi: Sri Satguru Publications.
An academic word-for-word translation with indication of Sanskrit grammar and roots for words. An excellent reference book for the serious student.

Desikachar, T.K.V. 1987. *Patañjali's Yogasūtras*. New Delhi: Affiliated East-West Press.
An interpretation rather than a direct translation, useful as an introduction.

Feuerstein, Georg. 1989. *The Yoga-Sūtra of Patañjali*. Rochester: Inner Traditions International.
A scholarly word-for-word translation, though some of the language can be obscure.

Hartranft, Chip. 2003. *The Yoga Sūtras of Patañjali*. Boston and London: Shambhala.
An interesting interpretation, which avoids using Sanskrit words and brings out strong links to Buddhist ideas and themes.

Moors, Frans. 2012. *Liberating Isolation: The Yogasūtra of Patañjali*. Chennai, India: Krishnamacharya Yoga Mandiram.
Another useful translation by one of Desikachar's senior students, which includes a word-for-word translation. Very user-friendly.

Prasada, Rama. 1912, 2007 reprint. *Patanjali's Yoga Sūtra*. New Delhi: Munshiram Manoharlal Publishers.
A scholarly and thorough translation including translations of Vyāsa and Vachaspati Mishra.

Hariharānanda, Swāmi. 1983. *Yoga Philosophy of Patañjali*. Albany: State University of New York.
Includes commentary of Vyāsa. Difficult to comprehend but one of the few serious translations of Vyāsa's commentary. Essential for serious students.

Related Books

Desikachar, T.K.V. 1995. *Heart of Yoga: Developing a Personal Practice*. Rochester: Inner Traditions.

– (eds. Mary Louise Skelton and Ross Carter). 1980. *Religiousness in Yoga*. Lanham, Maryland: University Press of America.

– 1982. *The Yoga of T. Krishnamacharya*. Chennai, India: Krishnamacharya Yoga Mandiram.

– 1998. *In Search of Mind*. New Delhi: Affiliated East-West Press.

– 1998. *Śrī Nāthamuni's Yogarahasya*. Chennai, India: Krishnamacharya Yoga Mandiram.

– 2000. *Yogayājñavalkya Samhitā*. Chennai, India: Krishnamacharya Yoga Mandiram.

Desikachar, T.K.V. with R.H. Craven. 1988. *Health, Healing & Beyond: Yoga and the Living Tradition of T. Krishnamacharya*. New York: Aperture Books.

Desikachar, T.K.V. and Neal Martyn. 2001. *What Are We Seeking?* Chennai, India: Krishnamacharya Yoga Mandiram.

Eliade, Mircea. 1958. Yoga: *Immortality and Freedom*. London: Arkana.

Feuerstein, Georg. 1989. *Yoga: The Technology of Ecstasy*. New York: TarcherPerigee/Penguin USA.

– 1998. *The Yoga Tradition*. Chino Valley, AZ: Hohm Press.

Goldberg, Elliot. 2016. *The Path of Modern Yoga: The History of an Embodied Spiritual Practice*. Rochester: Inner Traditions.

Harvey, Paul. 2001. *Yoga for Every Body*. London: Time-Life Books.

Hersnack, Peter. 2018. *The Living Breath: An Art of Yoga*. Art of Yoga.

Iyengar, B.K.S. 1964. *Light on Yoga: The Definitive Guide to Yoga Practice*. London: Allen & Unwin.

Kraftsow, Gary. 1999. *Yoga For Wellness*. New York: Penguin Books.

– 2002. *Yoga For Transformation*. New York: Penguin Books.

Larson, Gerald J. 1979. *Classical Sāmkhya*. New Delhi: Motilal Banarsidass.

Mallinson, James and Mark Singleton. 2017. *Roots of Yoga*. London: Penguin Classics.

Mohan, A.G. 1993. *Yoga for Body, Breath and Mind: A Guide to Personal Reintegration* Oregon: Rudra Press.

Mohan, A.G. and Ganesh Mohan. 2010. *Krishnamacharya: His Life and Teachings*. Boston and London: Shambala.

– 2013. *Yoga Yājñavalkya*. Chennai: Svastha.

– 2017. *Haṭha Yoga Pradīpikā*. Chennai: Svastha.

– 2015. *Yoga Reminder: Lightened Reflections*. Chennai: Svastha.

Mohan, A.G. and Indra Mohan. 2004. *Yoga Therapy: A Guide to the Therapeutic Use of Yoga and Ayurveda for Health and Fitness*. Boston and London: Shambhala.

Monier-Williams, M. 1899. *Sanskrit-English Dictionary*. Oxford: Oxford University Press.

Radhakrishnan, S. 1953, new edition 2006. *The Principal Upaniṣads*. New Delhi: HarperCollins India.

Ramaswami, Srivatsa. 2004. *The Complete Book of Vinyasa Yoga*. Boston: Marlow & Company.

– 2000. *Yoga for the Three Stages of Life: Developing Your Practice As an Art Form, a Physical Therapy, and a Guiding Philosophy*. Rochester: Inner Traditions.

Ramaswami, Srivatsa and David Hurwitz. 2006. *A Brief Introduction to Yoga Philosophy*. Boston: Marlow & Company.

Sargeant, Winthrop. 1984. *The Bhagavad Gītā*. Albany: State University of New York Press.

Singleton, Mark. 2010. *Yoga Body: The Origins of Modern Posture Practice*. Oxford & New York: Oxford University Press.

Svātmārāma. 1972. *The Haṭhayogapradīpikā*. Trans. Tookaram Tatya. Chennai: Adyar Library and Research Centre.

Acknowledgements

To all our many Kickstarter backers who contributed and who have waited so long, we offer our sincere thanks for your patience and your support:

Aimee Blackman, Becky Foyle, Sheila Reynolds, Cheryl Blamey and David Bennet, Kate Barnes, Amanda Oakes, Barbara Dancer, Michael Wegerer, Lisa Phillips, Ruth Gilmore, Leila Smith, Belinda Jobst, Jacqueline McGeever, Chris Preist, Liz Steward, Steve Welch, John Wace, Gillian Capps, Kathryn Van Howe, Sabine Dahn, Kirstie Rosser, Mike Brook, April Totham, Annie Wilson, Mark Singleton, Helen Sheppard, John Roy, Nicky Jacques, Pamela Cook, Zoe Herington, Miranda Bevis, Philip Copestake, Hugh Barford, Penny Phillips, Julie Taylor, Jonathan Paul, Connie Walsh, Pim Jackson, Rebecca Shah, Julian Fraser, Sara Bloxham, Dave and Lucy Tipper, John Malik, Brenda Hubbard, Valerie Young, Stephanie Mathews, Jacqueline Low, Dr Janet Anderson, Martin Brunsden, Sandra Lewis, Michelle Hebbron, Berit Lindholm, Sara Wills, Sandra Harvey, Linda Sharp, Bram Williams, Suzi Griffin, Becky Lewis, Jay and Em Goldmark, Beth Cox, Mrs Alexandra Soden, Marie Hudson, Caroline Hanks, Yvonne Sandison, Jill Chapman, Lisa Soede, Archie MacDonald, B. A. Guruswamy, Trudy Coulton, Sheila Baker, Elgin Heuerding, Anita Bulwer, Chantal Raffety & Gareth Williams, Kate Plummer, Debbie Charlett, Caroline Harris, Sue Chudley, Sophie Adams, Jen Musgrave, T.W. Chao, Jennifer Tennant, Jane Casey, Helena del Pino, Jane Harris, Lynne Scott, Rosie Paskins, Ann French, Paula O'Shagnessy, Kristy Stanley, Irena Hanman, Anne Smythe, Daisy Alegre-Cruz, Tom Kitching, Tara Hawes, Liz Lennon, Lynda Ryalls, Marion Lepetre, Sophie Rudolph, Mairead Flynn, Annie McDowall, Maria Ellerbeck, Su Bowler, Penny Cronyn, Peter Webber, Thomas Petit, Rosie Stephens, Liz Francis, Jane Elkins, Shital Pattani, Felicity Leigh, Cathy Salah, Bethan Walton, David Wilkinson, Sue Salmon, Rowan Pubble, Paul Moloney, Susan Cole, Helen Elger, Lesley Hay, Ben Wheatcroft, Jan Cumming, Deirdre Irwin, Katherine Biggs, Maggie Pollard, Tom Gaskell, Jane Southwell, Sue Gallagher, Lisa Smith, Colette Batterbee, Nicolas Nelissen, Sarah Cox, David Cary, Kath, Gibby Swaine, Rachel Done, Hilary Macrae, Susan Dick, Chiara Ghiron, Rosemary Phelan, Reuben Katz, Jodie Holdway, Cathie Pilgrim, Karen Waloschek, Kath Woods, Sharon Lovell, Rosemary Booker, Chloe Vernon, Mary Booker, Jose Kirby, Karolina Hryggr-Býr, Liz Woollard, Suzanne Spreadbury, Yvonne Cattermole, Jackie Dyson, Penelope Coomber, Mark Adams, Angela Roberts, Lesley Dever, Jane Tipping, Susan Neale, Keith Graham, Emily Foyle, Clara Lemon, Chloe Fremantle, Carolyn Norwich, Zana Mckenna, Gail Clarke, Rebecca Piesse, Caroline Arthur, Lesley Muir, Liz Lambert, Jane McLoughlin, Lucy Farr, Mary Evans, Sharon Hamilton, Cheryl Ormerod, Annie Durham, Margery Knowles, Sandra Webber, Lyn Barbour, Kate Blackmore, Claire Rigby, Annette Bauer, Erika Lyons, Becky Sperring, Cynthia Berman, Amanda Baxter, Veronica Moulder, Siobhan Brown, Jo McNeil, Angela Hendry, Tabitha Cohen, Kate Morris, Debbie Falchi, Rachel Heckbert, Noemi Franco, Matthew, Siobhan Rice, Heulwen L. James, Lynne Richardson, Linda Drewett, Judie Shore, Leigh Lamming, Sandy Parkin, Anika Grimm, Hilary Norman, Hilda Platje, Sabrina Tyus Hayes, Genevieve Shaw, Fiona Agombar, Mike Sheasby, Jacqui Storm, Penny Milne, Felicity O'Neill, Polly Rodgers, Susan Wall, Rachel Harding, Robert Winter, Liz Knott, Mike Young, Maryrose Loxley, Karthika Naïr, Sue Moon, Cheryl Kehyaian, Gill Boag-Munroe, Duncan Baldwin, Laura Blatchford, Caro Schiansky and Stephanie Phillips Morgan.

Ranju's sister, (the peerless) Anita Roy, has been project manager, liaison officer, cheerleader, editor, reader, prodder, agent, champion and roller of eyes-er. Thanks Anita for doing all this with such good humour and patience. We owe you so much – but your brother still won't let you win at table tennis.

Thanks to Martin and Zoë Hutton at Pinter & Martin for helping to midwife this book into the world. Our thanks also to Peter Turner at Red Wheel who has championed the book in the US, and has helped us to reach out to a far wider audience.

Knowing that the book is detailed, technical and quite dense, we also wanted it to look beautiful. We are grateful to Allan Sommerville who has done such a good job in keeping a feeling of spaciousness in the layout, and also to Charles Cox for his stunning calligraphy of the *devanāgarī* script which we have adapted and used at the beginning of each chapter. Thanks also to Olivia Fraser, whose beautiful watercolour painting adorns the UK edition front cover.

Ranju and Dave met each other on the same yoga retreat run by Paul Harvey in 1987. Since that time, we have shared the ups and downs, the ins and outs, the highs and the lows of our yoga journeys with many fellow teachers and students. To our yoga brothers and sisters – it's been great sharing and learning with you. In particular, our thanks to Mike Young, Chris Preist, Jenny Bullough, Hanne Gillespie, Sheila Baker, Eleanor Dawson, Hilary Norman and Steve Brandon. And of course, the many other of our fellow students who have travelled with us on the journey.

We started to work together as Sādhana Mālā in 2004, and over the years we have run many training courses, retreats and workshops. To all of the many students we have worked with in different situations, including our group classes and our 1-1 work, we offer our thanks. From each of you we have refined our understandings and developed our teachings.

Our initial teacher was Paul Harvey, who championed the teachings of Desikachar and Krishnamacharya when they were still virtually unknown in the UK in the 1980s. Paul has made a huge contribution to the understanding of yoga in the UK and he helped nurture and deepen our understandings. Through the 1990s we also worked with TKV Desikachar on a number of intensives, workshops and retreats.

We both met Peter Hersnack, another of Desikachar's early students, in 2004 and worked with him regularly until he passed away in 2016. Peter was a truly gifted teacher whose insights shone a new light on familiar ideas. He gave us permission to play, to explore and to look at things afresh – teachings, ideas, practices and even people.

As well as these three principle teachers, we have worked at various times with other teachers in this lineage including Srivatsa Ramaswami, Navtej Johar, R. Sriram, Sheela and Ravi Shankar, Sylviane Gianine and Frans Moors. We spent some very enjoyable time with AG Mohan on one of his visits to the UK and our discussions with him, although brief, had a big impact. To all of these teachers we offer our thanks and respect. Dave would also like to acknowledge his past teachers from the Buddhist tradition whose ideas continue to influence him profoundly, in particular Rob Preece, Rigdzin Shikpo and Shenpen Hookham.

Ranju would also like to thank his mum and dad, Hilary and Mihir Roy, who fostered a sense of curiosity and scepticism amidst a multicultural hotchpotch of Eastern/Western, scientific/arty, spiritual/secular, playful/serious. Without you, quite literally and for various reasons, this definitely would not have happened. And ever since he was conceived, Ranju's twin brother Sanjoy Roy has been there to compare, contrast, compete and communicate with. Sanj: I wouldn't me without you, and this book wouldn't have been this book. Ranju's Indian grandfather,

Sisir Kumar Roy, was the first person to give Ranju a book on yoga when he was fourteen. An enthusiastic practitioner until well into his 90s, he ignited Ranju's early interest in Indian spirituality: thanks, Dadu!

To Ranju's children Polly, Kiran and Rohan: thanks for listening to all my pontifications, laughing at my feeble jokes and keeping it real when it needs to be kept real. You all have contributed – in one way or another – to the ideas developed in the book.

Dave would like to thank everyone in his family for their forbearance and steady support over the years. In particular thanks to Duncan Reeves who encouraged us to write what would become our 'Funky Guru' pamphlets – which led us on a journey, culminating in this book.

And finally, to Lindy and Gail, our respective life partners. This project has taken so much time and energy on top of our already busy schedules; without you it just would not have happened. Gail once joked that she wondered whether she would ever see this book in her lifetime, as its birthing pains have taken a toll on us all. But, finally, it is here, and we are all still breathing, if a few years older and a little greyer for the process. To you both, who have given so much love and support, clarified our directions and given us the space to reflect, create and then write this book, we are forever indebted. Big love to you both.

Index